DIAMORPHINE

DIAMORPHINE

Its chemistry, pharmacology and clinical use

Edited by D. Bruce Scott, MD, FRCPE, FFARCS
Consultant Anaesthetist, Royal Infirmary, Edinburgh

This book has been commissioned by Evans Medical Limited as a service to the medical and pharmaceutical professions

WOODHEAD-FAULKNER
New York   London   Toronto   Sydney   Tokyo

Published by Woodhead-Faulkner Limited,
Simon & Schuster International Group,
Fitzwilliam House, 32 Trumpington Street,
Cambridge CB2 1QY, England
in association with Evans Medical Limited, Langhurst,
Horsham, West Sussex RH12 4QD, England.

First published 1988

© Evans Medical Limited 1988

British Library Cataloguing in Publication Data
Diamorphine.
Its chemistry, pharmacology and clinical use
  1. Man. Pain. Drug therapy. Heroin
  I. Scott, D. Bruce
  616'.0472

  ISBN 0-85941-381-0

Library of Congress Cataloging in Publication Data
Diamorphine
Its chemistry, pharmacology and clinical use.
  Includes index.
  1. Heroin—Therapeutic use—Testing. 2. Heroin—
Metabolism. 3. Pain—
Chemotherapy—Evaluation.
I. Scott, D. Bruce (Donald Bruce) [DNLM: 1. Diacetyl-
morphine—pharmacokinetics. 2. Diacetylmorphine—
pharmacology. 3. Diacetylmorphine—therapeutic use.
4. Pain—drug therapy. QV 92 D537]
RM666.H35D53 1988 616.86'3 88–5611
ISBN 0–85941–381–0

Designed by Andrew Shoolbred
Line drawings by Chris Walker
Typeset by Wyvern Typesetting Limited, Bristol
Printed in Great Britain by Anchor Brendon Limited, Tiptree, Essex

Contents

Contributors

Derek Doyle, OBE, FRCSE, FRCPE, FRCGP
Medical Director,
St Columba's Hospice,
Edinburgh.

Professor Christopher J. Hull, FFARCS
Professor of Anaesthesia,
University of Newcastle.

Honorary Consultant Anaesthesia,
Royal Infirmary,
Newcastle upon Tyne.

Leon Kaufman, MD, FFARCS
Consultant Anaesthetist,
University College Hospital,
London

Consultant Anaesthetist,
St Mark's Hospital,
London.

Senior Lecturer,
Faculty of Chemical Sciences,
University College London,
School of Medicine.

Henry A. S. Payne, BSc, PhD, C.Chem, MRSC
New Products Development Manager,
Macfarlan Smith Limited,
Edinburgh.

Alex T. Proudfoot, BSc, FRCPE
Consultant Physician,
Royal Infirmary,
Edinburgh.

Director,
Scottish Poisons Information Bureau.

J. Roy Robertson, MRCGP
General Practitioner,
Edinburgh.

D. Bruce Scott, MD, FRCPE, FFARCS
Consultant Anaesthetist,
Royal Infirmary,
Edinburgh.

Lloyd A. Stevens, BSc, PhD
Hazelton Medical Research Unit,
Springfield House,
Leeds.

Sue M. Tempest, B.Pharm, MPS
Pharmacist Medicines Research Unit,
Derbyshire Royal Infirmary.

Robert G. Twycross, MA, DM, FRCP
Consultant Physician,
The Churchill Hospital,
Headington,
Oxford.

Christina M. Wootton, BSc, Dip. Info. Sci.
Medical Division,
Glaxo Group Research Ltd,
Greenford,
Middlesex.

ROBERT G. TWYCROSS, MA, DM, FRCP

Foreword

In recent years, many doctors and their fellow health-care workers have become particularly concerned about pain relief. In relation to cancer, this is reflected in the development of Hospices and Palliative Care Services, notably in the United Kingdom, North America, New Zealand and Australia. There has also been a parallel development of Pain Clinics and Pain Relief Units. These are now to be found in most countries and are concerned with chronic pain of both non-malignant and malignant origin. National and regional Pain Societies have proliferated and, in 1987, the Fifth World Congress on Pain took place under the auspices of the International Association for the Study of Pain.

In severe acute pain and in chronic cancer pain, drug therapy remains the mainstay of management. A 1986 World Health Organization report, *Cancer Pain Relief*, stated: 'Relatively small amounts of inexpensive drugs suffice in the great majority of cases.' The particular importance of morphine was emphasised, and a strong plea was made for the ready availability of oral preparations of this time-honoured drug. Here, however, attention is focused on diamorphine (diacetylmorphine). As the alternative chemical name indicates, diamorphine is morphine plus two acetyl groups. Thus, the aim of this book is to show what these two groups do to morphine. It is the first attempt for many years to bring together current knowledge about diamorphine from a variety of disciplines. Those of us who have participated in any way in the development of this body of knowledge will recognise the book as an important contribution to its study.

Diamorphine has been a controversial drug since the early part of this century. It must therefore be stated unequivocally that, however fascinating it is to the scientist, and however attractive it may be to the addict, diamorphine has no unique properties as an analgesic. Pains can be divided into opioid-responsive and opioid-non-responsive; they cannot be divided into morphine-responsive and diamorphine-responsive. Pain that does not respond to morphine will not respond to diamorphine, and vice versa. On the other hand, diamorphine does possess distinct physicochemical properties which influence both its pharmacokinetic and its pharmacodynamic characteristics. This makes it an attractive alternative to morphine in a number of clinical settings. An understanding of these properties is necessary if diamorphine is to be placed appropriately in the therapeutic armamentarium.

D. BRUCE SCOTT, MD, FRCPE, FFARCS

Preface

There can be few drugs on which opinions differ so much as diamorphine, and few drugs which have been the source of more illogical thought and practice by those using it both medically and illegally.

Morphine, in the form of opium, has been the standard 'strong' analgesic for centuries. Because of its psychoactive properties it has also been used non-medically for just as long. The medical and non-medical use of psychotropic drugs seldom go hand in hand in terms of usage and popularity. Cocaine, which was widely used between 1884 and 1960 for local anaesthesia and in analgesic mixtures for the dying, has almost disappeared from medical practice at a time when there has been an enormous increase in its non-medical use.

Diamorphine, under its trade name Heroin, achieved popularity in medical practice during the first half of the twentieth century, being preferred to morphine for its greater potency and more rapid effect. Its illegal use only started on any scale in the 1920s. Because of the dangers of abuse and addiction, it was banned from medicinal use in the United States of America in 1924 and vigorous international pressure was brought to ban the drug universally. Almost all countries yielded to this pressure, with the exception of the United Kingdom and a few others. In countries in which it was banned, particularly the United States, its illegal use nevertheless increased alarmingly. It virtually totally replaced morphine as a 'street' drug, probably because its high solubility allowed the easy intravenous injection of the huge doses used by addicts.

Where it is still available for medical use, it remains more popular than morphine, particularly in the relief of pain in the terminally ill. The reasons given for this preference are many and varied. However, it has to be admitted that, like many old drugs, the scientific basis for claims for and against its use are questionable. In particular, its position *vis à vis* morphine has been studied properly in very few instances. Given that diamorphine is metabolised to monoacetyl morphine and morphine itself, it is surprising that it is different. When given orally, it is not unreasonable to consider it as a prodrug of morphine. However, it is more potent and quicker acting than morphine when given parenterally and it differs in important physicochemical properties affecting its pharmacokinetics and dynamics.

It may be unfortunate but it is nevertheless true, that the addictive properties of the opioids have greatly influenced the attitude of those using them medically, leading to suboptimal use. Fear that patients, given these drugs to relieve pain, would become addicted and dependent has meant that vast numbers of those suffering even severe pain are denied adequate analgesia. Where they are prescribed, dosage is often too small or administration too infrequent, therefore recourse to less effective analgesics is too readily taken. Both doctors and nurses are guilty of this irrational attitude. The problem of creating addiction in treating acute pain is so small as to be infinitesimal. Even with terminal cancer pain, which may last months or years, diamorphine or morphine have of themselves hardly ever been associated with physical or mental deterioration. We are grateful to our colleagues in the hospice movement working with the terminally ill, for showing how these patients can derive the maximum benefit without fear of addiction, if the drugs are used rationally.

In recent years, the use of intraspinal opioids has become popular, both for acute and chronic pain. The physicochemical properties of diamorphine could make it an ideal drug for this purpose.

As diamorphine remains a popular medical drug wherever it is legally available, it was thought that an up to date account of its chemistry, pharmacology and clinical use would be of value. In addition, the problems of overdosage and addiction have been addressed. While the prime interest of this book is in diamorphine, the clinical use of opioids generally is described where relevant. The word 'opioid' (meaning opium-like, usually referring to synthetic drugs) has been generally preferred in the text to 'opiate' (meaning derived from opium). This terminology leaves the whole group of drugs without a common title. While every effort has been made to be consistent, this has not been possible in every instance. Throughout the book, the name 'diamorphine' has been used and not 'heroin' as the latter was its original trade name; diamorphine being its correct generic title. The authors hope that this monograph will be of use as a reference book to all those scientists and clinicians who have an interest in this important drug.

HENRY A. S. PAYNE, BSc, PhD, C. Chem, MRSC
SUE M. TEMPEST, B. Pharm, MPS

1 The chemistry and pharmacy of diamorphine

Structure

Diamorphine (II), or diacetylmorphine, is one of many hundreds of opiate derivatives which have been synthesised from morphine (I). It is one of the lower members of a series of morphine diesters and the only one to achieve any importance. Diamorphine is derived from morphine by replacing the hydroxylic hydrogens on the phenolic oxygen at position 3, and the alcoholic oxygen at position 6, by acetyl groups. As might be expected, the presence of two acetyl substituents affects both the physical and chemical properties of the molecule.

It is informative to compare the structure of diamorphine (II) with that of morphine (I) and other morphine derivatives (see Fig. 1.1), some of which are analgesics with various potencies, e.g. oxymorphone (IX), hydromorphone (VII) and codeine (IV), some antitussives, e.g. ethylmorphine (V) and pholcodine (VI), and some narcotic antagonists, for example, naloxone (VIII) and nalorphine (X). The structure of the principal degradation product of diamorphine, i.e., 6-O-acetylmorphine (III), is also shown.

As described above, diamorphine differs from morphine by the presence of two acetyl groups. In morphine, the 3-hydroxyl group attached to a benzenoid ring is phenolic, that is, it is sufficiently acidic to dissolve in alkaline or strongly basic solutions. The 6-hydroxyl group in the lower ring behaves as a cyclic alcohol. The difference in nature of these two hydroxyl groups accounts for the difference in the rate of hydrolysis of

1

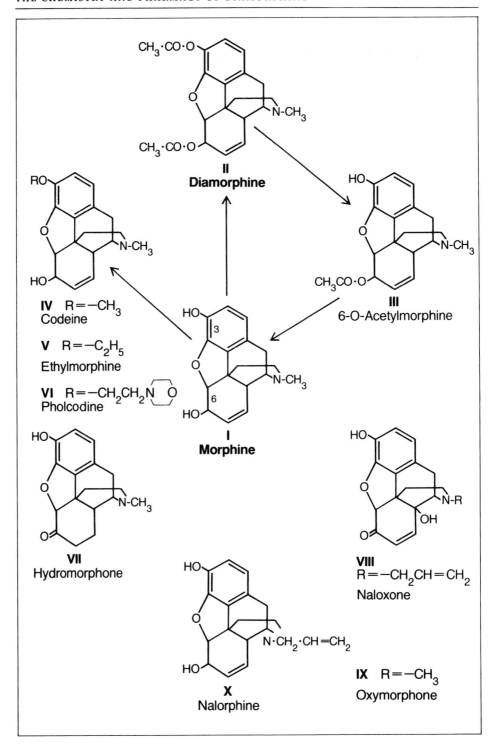

Fig. 1.1 Morphine and other opiate derivatives.

the acetyl groups in diamorphine. The presence of the two hydroxyl groups in morphine tends to decrease its lipid solubility, whereas the two acetyl groups in diamorphine tend to increase it. In 6-O-acetylmorphine, the initial degradation product of diamorphine, the 3-acetyl group, has been lost by hydrolysis leaving a free phenolic group and giving a molecule intermediate in character between that of morphine and diamorphine. Another possible monoacetyl derivative is 3-O-acetylmorphine. There have been a number of reports of its preparation, but it is doubtful whether it has ever been isolated in a pure form. If it is a decomposition product of diamorphine, it does not play a major part and will not be considered further.

The structure of diamorphine may also be compared with the structures of other potent opiate analgesics such as hydromorphone (VII) and oxymorphone (IX). These two molecules have more affinity with morphine than with diamorphine and only differ from each other by the presence of a hydroxyl group in the 14-position of oxymorphone. They differ from morphine at position 6 where the morphine hydroxyl is replaced by a carbonyl group. The presence of a carbonyl group does appear to modify one property of the molecule – the water solubility of the hydrochloride salt which, in each case, is very much greater than that of morphine hydrochloride. The presence of a free phenolic group at the 6-position would appear to be common to all these powerful analgesics except for diamorphine. Why is diamorphine different? The difference may only be apparent since there is good evidence to show that diamorphine undergoes rapid breakdown in the bloodstream to give 6-O-acetylmorphine which, of course, boasts a free phenolic group, and that it is this degradation product which is the active species.

The structure/activity relationship, however, must not be oversimplified, nor extrapolated too far, as other groups on the morphine skeleton are also important. Naloxone (VIII) has a free phenolic group at position 3 and differs only from oxymorphone by the presence of an allyl (—$CH_2CH = CH_2$ group instead of a methyl (—CH_3) group on the nitrogen at position 17. Naloxone is a potent narcotic antagonist. Nalorphine (X), which bears the same relationship to morphine as naloxone does to oxymorphone, with an allyl rather than a methyl substituent on the nitrogen, also displays antagonist properties.

The ease with which the 3-acetyl group in diamorphine is lost may be contrasted with the difficulty encountered in removing a 3-methyl ether group as found in codeine (IV). Ether linkages are extremely stable and require drastic conditions to cleave them. This stability no doubt modifies the analgesic property of the molecule which is very much less than that of morphine.

3

Physical properties

In discussing the physical properties of diamorphine we must consider both the free base and the hydrochloride salt as separate entities. Salt formation greatly increases the water solubility of almost all opiate drugs thereby simplifying the problem of administering them. Some of the properties of the principal opiates and their hydrochloride salts are shown in Table 1.1.

Table 1.1 Physical properties of opiate derivatives.

OPIATE DERIVATIVE	ANHYDROUS MOLECULAR WEIGHT	MELTING POINT °C	SOLUBILITY IN WATER	SOLUBILITY IN ETHANOL
6-O-acetylmorphine base	327.4	192	40 ml	–
6-O-acetylmorphine hydrochloride	363.8	298	ss	–
Codeine base	299.4	155	120 ml	2 ml
Codeine hydrochloride	335.9	264	20 ml	180 ml
Diamorphine base	369.4	173	1,200 ml	33 ml
Diamorphine hydrochloride	405.9	243[1]	1.6 ml	12 ml
Hydromorphone base	285.3	266	i	s
Hydromorphone hydrochloride	321.8	280	3 ml	100 ml (90%)
Morphine base	285.8	254	5,000 ml	250 ml
Morphine hydrochloride	322.3	200	24 ml	100 ml
Morphine sulphate	334.4[2]	250	21 ml	1,000 ml
Oxymorphone	301.3	248	i	s
Oxymorphone hydrochloride	337.8	300	4 ml	100 ml
Naloxone hydrochloride	363.8	200	s	ss

s = soluble
ss = slightly soluble
i = insoluble
solubilities = volume of solvent to dissolve 1 gm

(1) on anyhydrous material
(2) sulphate is a dibasic anion. The molecular weight given is equivalent to one morphine molecule: actual molecular weight is 668.8

Diamorphine base is a colourless, odourless solid with a bitter taste which emits an acetic odour on exposure to damp air and slowly turns pink. The melting point lies between that of codeine and 6-O-acetylmorphine but is much lower than that of morphine. The free base exits in two crystalline forms: form 1, rods and oblique plates; form 2, spherulites. The latter melts at 5°C lower, is less stable than the former and can be converted back into form 1. The base is essentially insoluble in water but dissolves in ethanol. It is more soluble in benzene (1 g in 8 ml) and in chloroform (1 g in 1.5 ml) but is only slightly soluble in ether (1 g in 100 ml).

Diamorphine hydrochloride is likewise a colourless, odourless crystalline solid with a bitter taste. It decomposes, more slowly than the base, in the presence of damp air to give an acetic odour. It can exist both as the anhydrous salt or more commonly as the stable monohydrate, the anhydrous salt melting ten degrees higher than the hydrate. The hydrochloride is very soluble in water and is also readily soluble in ethanol. It is insoluble in benzene and ether but like the base is soluble in chloroform (1 g in 1.6 ml). In dilute solution it is completely dissociated, and its conductivity is comparable to a strong binary electrolyte. The pH of an 0.01 molar solution is 5.2 and its pKa at 23°C is 7.63.

The structures of both base and hydrochloride have been confirmed by infra-red, nuclear magnetic resonance and mass spectroscopy. Separation of diamorphine from other opiates may be effected by the standard techniques of thin layer, gas liquid, and high-performance liquid chromatography.

On a molecular, three-dimensional level, diamorphine exhibits a T-configuration typical of many of the natural members of the morphine alkaloid series (see Fig. 1.2).

Diamorphine hydrochloride has a high anhydrous molecular weight compared with some of the other potent analgesics (see Table 1.1). This is due entirely to the contribution from the two acetyl groups. The melting points of the hydrochlorides are all high, though diamorphine hydrochloride is one of the lowest, apart from morphine. Their solubilities in water are all comparable, again with the exception of morphine.

Chemical properties

The chemical breakdown of diamorphine into acetic acid and 6-O-acetylmorphine will be dealt with in the Stability section (see page 7).

Diamorphine is a strong base capable of forming salts with many acids. The hydrochloride, however, is the only major salt to have been fully described in the literature. Diamorphine undergoes a number of

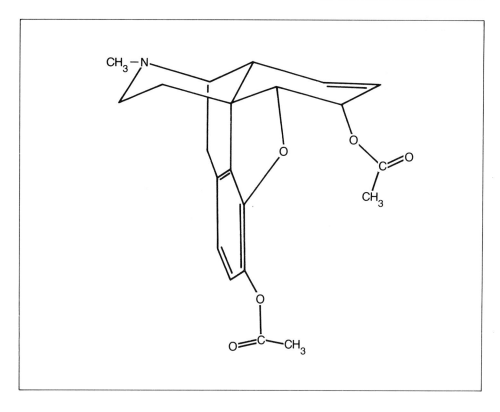

Fig. 1.2 Three-dimensional structure of diamorphine.

reactions typical of the main series of opiate alkaloids. It is readily hydrogenated over a precious metal catalyst to give dihydrodiamorphine, also a potent analgesic. With bromine water it brominates in the 1-position to give 1-bromodiamorphine. In the reaction with hydrogen peroxide, the principal product is 6-O-acetylmorphine N-oxide, the acetyl group at position 3 being lost. Cyanogen bromide, a reagent used for removing the methyl group from the nitrogen at position 17, undergoes a reaction with diamorphine to give N-cyanonordiamorphine. This in turn can be converted into normorphine by the hydrolysis of both the cyano and acetyl groups, and so provides a route to nalorphine and other morphine derivatives in which the N-methyl group is replaced by another substituent.

Before the days of rapid analysis by the modern chromatographic techniques, diamorphine could be identified by, or distinguished from, morphine by a series of colour tests with readily-available reagents. Some of these tests are listed in Table 1.2.

Table 1.2 Colour reactions of diamorphine and its degradation products.

TEST REAGENT	MORPHINE	6-O-ACETYLMORPHINE	DIAMORPHINE
Concentrated nitric acid	Orange red	Red→blue	Yellow→bluish green→yellow
Ferric chloride and potassium ferricyanide	Bluish green	Blue colour	Blue colour on heating
Erdmann's Test[1]	Carmine	–	Pale yellow
Marquis' Test[2]	Purple→ violet	Purple	Red-violet→ violet
Ammonium molybdate	Purple→ blue→ light green	Violet	As morphine
Ammonium vanadate	Blue-grey	–	Very faint blue-grey
Potassium iodate, sulphuric acid, ammonia	Black	Yellow	No colour in cold

(1) Soldium hypochlorite and concentrated sulphuric acid

(2) Formaldehyde and concentrated sulphuric acid

Stability and compatibility

Diamorphine – drug substance

In a recent study, the stability of solid diamorphine hydrochloride was examined at ambient temperature and at 37 °C. The assay was carried out by high-performance liquid chromatography which measured the amounts of diamorphine and its two degradation products directly. Samples had been stored for up to two years at room temperature in the dark. The content of 6-O-acetylmorphine varied from 0.46 to 1.44% and of morphine from zero to 0.03%. On storage at 37 °C over a nine-month period, there was a slight moisture loss and the melting point was lowered marginally, but it remained within specification. The 6-O-acetylmorphine content was less than 1% and the morphine was only just detectable. It is clear that under suitable storage conditions pure diamorphine hydrochloride remains stable. Some indication of the stability of solid diamorphine base was given when a sample stored at ambient temperature for over 25 years was found to be almost 95% pure.

The stability of crystalline hydrate and anhydrous forms of the salt have been compared and differ only slightly. In practice the freeze-dried form is used and satisfactory stability is achieved with moisture levels of less than 3%.

Aqueous solution

Aqueous solutions of diamorphine hydrochloride are much less stable than solutions of morphine or codeine salts. Hydrolysis of the 3-acetyl group takes place both in the dark and in the cold. The 6-acetyl group also hydrolyses slowly to give morphine. It is therefore impractical to store solutions of diamorphine. Heating also decomposes solutions and it has been shown that the decomposition rate increases uniformly with increasing temperature. On exposure to daylight, an unbuffered 1% solution decomposes completely in one month. However, there are other reports in which incomplete conditions of storage are given, which indicate only 50% decomposition of a diamorphine solution in two years.

Hydrolysis is rapid but not necessarily complete under alkaline or acidic conditions. The most stable pH range would appear to be 4–5 in the presence of a phosphate buffer. The alkalinity of the glass may also be a contributing factor in the decomposition of solutions either directly or by some surface catalytic effect.

Diamorphine in saline

A major problem in determining the stability of diamorphine in solution has been the lack of a suitable specific assay for the acetylmorphines and morphine, which appear in stored diamorphine solutions. Neither quantitative thin layer chromatography (TLC) nor gas liquid chromatography (GLC) were satisfactory. With the development of high-performance liquid chromatography (HPLC) several methods were devised. Beaumont's method (Beaumont, 1982; Allwood, 1984; Regnard et al., 1986), using an ion-pairing agent, is particularly suitable, separating and quantifying diamorphine, 6-O-acetylmorphine and morphine without the necessity for prior extraction or dilution.

The time for 10% of a 1 mg/ml diamorphine solution at varying pH to degrade to 6-O-acetylmorphine was calculated ($T_{90\%}$). $T_{90\%}$ is generally accepted as the basis of the shelf life of pharmaceutical products. The results show that the maximum stability of diamorphine at room temperature is achieved at a pH 3.8–4.4 (ionic strength 0.5 M) in chloroform water. Very small increases in ionic strength give very large decreases in shelf life, and have a far greater effect than does pH on stability. Maximum shelf life is achieved when no buffer is present. The $T_{90\%}$ of a 1 mg/ml solution of diamorphine in chloroform water, pH 6.3–6.9, is approximately one month.

Although the use of morphine or diamorphine in chloroform water is now accepted as the preferred method for oral administration of these opiates in solution, some clinicians persist in the use of more traditional mixtures.

The Act-a-pump is a relatively new portable infusion device incorporating a 75 ml disposable reservoir which can deliver solutions at flow rates varying from 2–110 ml/24 hours. It can be set to run for up to 37 days without priming, thus necessitating the use of concentrated solutions of diamorphine (Jones and Hanks 1986; Jones *et al.*, 1985). Using high performance liquid chromatography (ultraviolet detection at 210 nm), Hanks *et al.* have since shown a concentration and temperature-dependent degradation of diamorphine with a corresponding increase in levels of 6-O-acetylmorphine and morphine (see Table 1.3).

Theoretically, it is possible to run the Act-a-pump over one month, but in clinical practice this is unlikely to exceed 14 days. 'The analgesic potency of the degradation product 6-O-acetylmorphine is thought to be approximately equipotent with diamorphine (Wright and Barbour, 1935), but a definitive clinical study has not been reported.' The clinical consequences of the degradation of diamorphine to 6-O-acetylmorphine under the conditions described would therefore be minimal. Further decomposition to morphine is sufficiently slow to be of little consequence.

Stability of diamorphine/saline solutions

The *British Pharmaceutical Codex* (11th edition, 1979) states that: 'Sodium chloride precipitates diamorphine from solutions and is not suitable for adjusting the tonicity of solutions'. However, recent work has challenged this statement (Page and Hudson, 1982; Kirk and Hain, 1985). Solutions of

Table 1.3 Percentage degradation of diamorphine in aqueous solution.

	21 °C		37 °C	
	1 mg/ml	250 mg/ml	1 mg/ml	250 mg/ml
Day 7	0.5	7.9	10.0	35.2
Day 14	2.7	8.5	13.0	54.5
Day 28	5.7	7.3	19.9	66.0
Day 42	10.6	11.0	32.6	85.8

diamorphine hydrochloride 0.05 to 5% w/v in sodium chloride injection BP of varying pH, and in citro-phosphate buffer pH 6.6, were observed for signs of precipitation over several days. The pH of each solution was checked before and after the addition of diamorphine hydrochloride, as well as at the end of the standing period. No visible precipitate was observed in the unbuffered solutions which all had a pH less than 6. Precipitation did occur in solutions buffered to 6.6 when the concentration of diamorphine hydrochloride was 0.5% w/v. Precipitation occurred at 2 hours (5% w/v) and 3 days (0.5% w/v) respectively. Thus it would appear that the addition of diamorphine hydrochloride to isotonic saline lowers the pH sufficiently to ensure that the solute remains in solution.

Following this paper, Martindale's *Extra Pharmacopoeia* (28th edition, 1982), stated: 'Sodium chloride may precipitate diamorphine from concentrated solutions at a pH above 5.5.'

The second study observed no precipitation after 24 hours of solutions of 0.02, 0.1, 0.2, 0.4% w/v diamorphine hydrochloride in sodium chloride solutions of 0.9, 1.8, 3.6, 7.2% w/v kept at 23 °C. The pH of each solution up to a diamorphine concentration of 0.2% was between 6.05 and 6.6, and of the 0.4% solutions between 5.65 and 5.9.

A further experiment with diamorphine hydrochloride 5% w/v in sodium chloride 0.9% w/v at pH 4.9 and 6.6 showed no sign of precipitation at the lower pH but at pH 6.6, needle-like crystals were observed after 24 hours.

Compatibility and stability of diamorphine/antiemetic mixtures

Some patients who require diamorphine for pain relief have intractable vomiting. The use of battery-operated syringe drivers to deliver diamorphine by continuous subcutaneous infusion circumvents the need for repeated 4-hourly injections. Antiemetics are often added to diamorphine solutions, though this is not required routinely (see page 77) as the antiemetic may be prescribed separately in those patients requiring them. Because these mixtures may be prepared some time in advance, their stability must be assessed. A number of antiemetics have been investigated in combination with varying concentrations of diamorphine. Some of these are listed below. Stability data obtained using one source of preparation may not always apply to medicaments obtained from other sources.

Diamorphine hydrochloride and cyclizine lactate

Cyclizine/diamorphine mixtures spanning a range of concentrations have been stored in the dark at room temperature and at 4, 21 and 32 °C. After 24 hours each sample was visually checked for discolouration, crystallisation and precipitation. The effect of adding lactate to the diamorphine/cyclizine mixtures is to keep cyclizine in solution up to a concentration of 30 mg/ml; (the concentration of diamorphine ranged up to 100 mg/ml). However, the low pH of the resulting solution means that it is of little practical value as it would most certainly cause irritation at the injection site.

Regnard and co-workers (1986) showed that cyclizine/diamorphine mixtures remain clear when the cyclizine concentration is below 10 mg/ml. As the concentration approaches 10–20 mg/ml, crystals of varying size and number form, and above 25 mg/ml, precipitation is likely, especially when the concentration of diamorphine also exceeds 25 mg/ml. Combinations of cyclizine and diamorphine in syringe drivers therefore may not be advisable.

Diamorphine hydrochloride and haloperidol
Solutions containing a final concentration of haloperidol greater than 1 mg/ml precipitate immediately. At 1 mg/ml crystals are seen after 7 days with a 58% loss of antiemetic. Combinations of haloperidol and diamorphine in syringe drivers therefore may also not be advisable.

Diamorphine hydrochloride and hyoscine
Both the butylbromide and the hydrobromide salts of hyoscine appear to be compatible with diamorphine at the concentrations tested.

Diamorphine hydrochloride and metoclopramide
Solutions of diamorphine and metoclopramide at the concentrations tested appear to have acceptable stability with regard to diamorphine content. However, slight discolouration occurs after 7 days. Loss in assayable metoclopramide is accompanied by a drop in the pH of the solution from 3.5 to 2.3, together with a clear metoclopramide degradation peak. Therefore if solutions of diamorphine and metoclopramide are to be used in syringe drivers they should be closely observed for signs of degradation.

Diamorphine hydrochloride and prochlorperazine mesylate
Solutions of diamorphine and prochlorperazine at the concentrations tested appear to have acceptable stability with regard to diamorphine content. However, prochlorperazine content has not been assayed, and in common with other phenothiazines, it causes irritation to subcutaneous tissues. In the United Kingdom it is not licensed to be given by this route.

Diamorphine hydrochloride and methotrimeprazine
Diamorphine appears to be stable in the presence of methotrimeprazine.

Formulations of diamorphine

Diamorphine tablets

Diamorphine hydrochloride 10 mg (for oral administration).

Diamorphine injection

Freeze-dried powder of diamorphine hydrochloride for reconstitution; 5 mg, 10 mg, 30 mg, 100 mg, 500 mg. Freeze-drying is a suitable method for preparing the parenteral preparation; as drying takes place at very low temperatures, hydrolysis is minimised. The solution of diamorphine is placed in ampoules and immediately transferred to a freeze drier where silicone fluid circulates at a temperature of $-60\,°C$. The final product is a network of solid occupying the same volume as the original solution. Thus, there is no case-hardening and the product is light and porous, which ensures ready solubility. The final product has a shelf life of three years.

Diamorphine hydrochloride is extremely soluble in water, 1 gm dissolving in 1.6 ml water at 25 °C. This means that only very small volumes of solution need to be injected, which is often advantageous in cachexic patients or when large doses need to be given.

Diamorphine solutions

A simple elixir of diamorphine in chloroform water is now preferred to traditional compound elixirs. It is normal practice to adjust the formulation so that each unit dose is contained in 5 or 10 ml. The formulae for some traditional compound elixirs containing cocaine and alcohol are no longer given in the *British National Formulary*. Their use is illogical and should be condemned (see page 73).

Diamorphine Linctus BPC

Diamorphine hydrochloride	3.00 mg
Compound Tartrazine solution	0.06 ml
Glycerol	1.25 ml
Oxymel	1.25 ml
Syrup	to 5.00 ml

It should be freshly prepared.

Diamorphine suppositories

These suppositories in varying strengths are made, on request, in a number of institutions in the United Kingdom. Witepsol is the usual base employed. No stability data is available.

Legal status of diamorphine prescriptions in the United Kingdom

Diamorphine and its salts are subject to the prescription requirements of the Misuse of Drugs Regulations 1973 and are described as 'Controlled Drugs' sometimes denoted by the symbol CD.

Prescriptions must be signed and dated by the prescriber. They must give his address and be in his own handwriting using indelible ink. In addition a prescription must state the following:

1. The name and address of the patient.
2. The form and, where appropriate, the strength of the preparation.
3. The total quantity of the drug or preparation, or the number of dose units; in both words and figures.
4. The dose. A prescription is valid for 13 weeks from the date stated thereon. Repeat prescriptions are not permitted. However, a prescription for a controlled drug (CD) may request that the medication be dispensed in instalments. The amount for each instalment and the intervals to be observed must be specified.

It is an offence for a doctor to issue an incomplete prescription for a CD and for a pharmacist to dispense it unless all the information required by law is present on the prescription. Forms are valid for supply on one occasion only.

The Misuse of Drugs Act 1971 prohibits certain activities in relation to CDs, in particular their manufacture, supply and possession. The penalties applicable to offences involving the different drugs are divided into three classes according to the harmfulness attributable to a drug when it is misused. Diamorphine is a class A type drug.

The Misuse of Drugs (Notification and Supply to Addicts) Regulations 1973 require that a medical practitioner must notify in writing the Chief Medical Officer, Drugs Branch, Queen Anne's Gate, London SW1H 9AT, of any person he considers or suspects is addicted to diamorphine. Written notification must be made within seven days of first becoming aware that the patient may be an addict.

The regulations also state that only medical practitioners who hold a special licence issued by the Home Secretary may prescribe diamorphine, dipipanone (Diconal) or cocaine for addicts. Other practitioners must refer their opioid-dependent patients to a treatment centre. Staff from the treatment centre normally introduce the addict to a particular pharmacist who has agreed to dispense for the patient. Subsequent prescriptions will be sent from the centre to the pharmacist by post. A request for alterations in the method of supply made by the addict must be agreed to by the treatment centre.

Medical practitioners are permitted to prescribe diamorphine for the relief of pain due to organic disease or injury without the use of a special licence.

References

Allwood, M. C., (1984), 'Diamorphine mixed with antiemetic drugs in plastic syringes', *British Journal of Pharmaceutical Practice*, **6**, 88.

Beaumont, I. M., (1982), 'A stability study of aqueous solutions of diamorphine and morphine using High-Performance Liquid Chromatography', *Proceedings of the Analytical Division of the Royal Society of Chemistry*, p. 129.

Bentley, K. W., *The Chemistry of Morphine Alkaloids*, (1954), (Oxford, Oxford University Press).

The British National Formulary, Number 14 (1987) (London, British Medical Association and the Pharmaceutical Press).

The British Pharmaceutical Codex (1973) (London, The Pharmaceutical Press).

Clarke, E. G. C., *Isolation and Identification of Drugs*, (1986), (London, The Pharmaceutical Press).

Jones, V. A., Hoskin, P. J., Omar, O. A., Johnson, A., Hanks, G. W. and Turner, P., (1986), 'Diamorphine stability in aqueous solution for subcutaneous infusion', *Abstracts of the British Pharmacological Society Meeting, 1986*, p. 66.

Jones, V. A. and Hanks, G. W., (1986), 'New portable infusion pump for prolonged subcutaneous administration of opioid analgesics in patients with advanced cancer', *British Medical Journal*, **292**, 1,496.

Jones, V. A., Murphy, A. and Hanks, G. W., (1985), 'Solubility of diamorphine', *Pharmaceutical Journal*, **235**, 426.

Kirk, B. and Hain, W. R., (1985), 'Diamorphine injection BP incompatibility', *Pharmaceutical Journal*, **235**, 171.

Martindale, (1982) *The Extra Pharmacopoeia*, Reynolds, J. E. F. (ed), (London, The Pharmaceutical Press, 28th edition).

The Merck Index, (1983), Merck & Co. Inc., (Rahway, NJ, USA, 10th edition).

Page, J. and Hudson, S., (1982), 'Diamorphine hydrochloride compatibility with saline', *Pharmaceutical Journal*, **228**, 238.

The Pharmaceutical Codex (1979), (London, The Pharmaceutical Press, 11th edition).

Regnard, C., Pashley, S. and Westrope, F., (1986), 'Antiemetic/diamorphine mixture compatability in infusion pumps', *British Journal of Pharmaceutical Practice*, **8**, 218.

Small, L. F., and Lutz, R. E., 'Chemistry of the Opium Alkaloids' (Supplement No. 103 to the Public Heath Reports) (1932) Washington.

LLOYD A. STEVENS, BSc, PhD

CHRISTINA M. WOOTTON, BSc, Dip. Info. Sci.

2 The pharmacokinetic properties of diamorphine

When a drug is prescribed by a clinician and taken by a patient, the primary objective is to produce a pharmacodynamic response that is effective in treating or alleviating the symptoms of a particular disease. However, several processes occur between the administration of the dose and the appearance of the desired therapeutic effect. These are illustrated in Fig. 2.1 which shows that absorption, distribution, metabolism and excretion are the major pharmacokinetic properties of a drug which influence the time course, and maybe the intensity, of the pharmaco-dynamic response. Drugs are usually administered to the body by the most convenient route that satisfies the therapeutic needs. Consequently it is not surprising to find that opiates such as diamorphine have been given intravenously, intramuscularly, orally and directly into the spinal canal to produce systemic or local effects as the situation requires.

The shape of the plasma drug concentration versus time curve will depend therefore on the following factors:
1. Route of administration.
2. Dosage form.
3. Dosage regimen.
4. Release of the drug from its formulation.
5. Absorption from the site of administration.
6. Distribution via the blood into organs and tissues of the body.
7. Routes and rates of metabolic transformation.
8. Routes and rates of excretion.
9. Alteration of any of the above by the disease state or age of the patient.

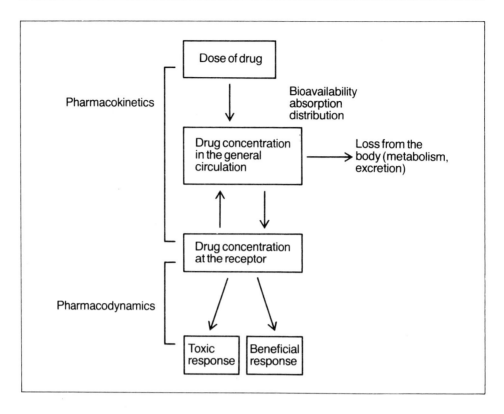

Fig. 2.1 Diagrammatic view of the relationship between the pharmacokinetics and pharmacodynamic properties of a drug.

The relative contribution of any of these factors is often determined by the physicochemical properties of the drug. These include, solubility, stability, partition coefficient, dissociation constant (pKa), lipophilicity and crystal morphology among others. The onset, duration and intensity of the pharmacodynamic response of a drug are therefore influenced as much by the biopharmaceutical properties of the formulation, and the pharmacokinetic properties of the drug, as they are by its intrinsic pharmacological behaviour. Moreover, if metabolic transformation results in the production of a pharmacologically active metabolite(s), the overall pharmacodynamic response would be influenced by the pharmacokinetic and pharmacological properties of that metabolite(s) in addition to those of the parent drug. This is particularly so where the metabolites have physicochemical and pharmacokinetic properties which are significantly distinct from those of the parent drug.

This chapter will review the pharmacokinetics of diamorphine in animals and man. Where possible the pharmacokinetics of diamorphine will be contrasted with those of its major metabolite(s) in an attempt to explain differences in their pharmacodynamic responses. The relationship between the route of diamorphine administration and the pharmaco-dynamic response will be highlighted. The influence of diamorphine on the action of other drugs, and vice versa, where the interaction is reported to have a pharmacokinetic basis, will also be discussed.

The ability to describe the pharmacokinetic properties of a drug depends entirely upon an ability to detect and measure the drug in biological fluids. Since specific and sensitive methods of drug analysis are central to any pharmacokinetic evaluation they will also be briefly reviewed in this chapter. As the qualitative identification techniques employed for forensic purposes are beyond the scope of this review, those interested are referred to review articles by Dutt, 1984; Harwood, 1974; Gorodetzky *et al.*, 1974; Hays *et al.*, 1973; Gough and Baker, 1983, and WHO report No. 556, 1974, among others. For previously published reviews on diamorphine disposition see Way and Adler, 1962; Boerner *et al.*, 1975; Misra, 1978, and Sawynok, 1986.

Details of all these publications are given in the Reference section at the end of this chapter (pages 38–43).

Physicochemical properties relevant to diamorphine and morphine pharmacokinetics

Absorption, distribution and elimination of drugs involves transfer of the drug molecules across various membranes such as the gastrointestinal epithelium, hepatocytes within the liver, renal tubular epithelia, blood-brain barrier and the placental membrane among others. The most common mechanism by which the majority of drugs cross membranes is passive diffusion, and the rate at which drug molecules transfer across biological membranes is a function of the concentration-gradient across the membrane, its surface area, and the ability of the drug to partition into the membrane. As far as drug molecules are concerned, biological mem-branes behave as if they are simple lipid barriers. Therefore only lipid soluble drugs or lipid soluble forms of a drug will diffuse freely across these membranes. Molecules such as diamorphine, 6-O-acetylmorphine and morphine are electrolytes and will appear in solution as ionised and nonionised forms. The nonionised form of these drugs is more lipid soluble than the ionised form. The degree of ionisation is determined by the dissociation constant of the drug (pKa) and the pH of the biological fluid. This relationship between drug pKa, lipid solubility, partitioning ability and diffusion across membranes is commonly known as the 'pH-partition hypothesis'. An index of lipid solubility is given by the partition coefficient which is a measure of the relative distribution of a drug between an aqueous phase (usually buffer at pH 7.4) and an organic phase (usually octanol, or chloroform).

Given a knowledge of the pKa and partition coefficient of diamorphine and morphine it is possible to compare their ability to transfer from one body fluid, e.g., plasma, into another, e.g., spinal fluid. A consideration of these variables (Table 2.1), particularly the much greater lipid solubility of diamorphine, leads to the assumption that diamorphine is more readily transferred across membranes than morphine, and presumably 6-O-acetylmorphine. This conclusion, based on physicochemical considerations alone has been substantiated by absorption, distribution and elimination studies in animals and man.

Pharmacokinetics of diamorphine after administration by various routes

Absorption describes the rate and extent to which a drug moves from its site of administration to its site of measurement (usually systemic circulation). This definition can be equally applied to oral, intramuscular, subcutaneous, inhaled, epidural, and intrathecal administration of diamorphine.

Subcutaneous

The pharmacological effects of morphine and diamorphine have been used in early studies as an index of absorption after subcutaneous administration to laboratory animals and man.

The higher aqueous solubility of diamorphine over that of morphine (Table 2.1) has facilitated chronic subcutaneous administration in patients unable to take the analgesic orally. Although no measurements of opiate levels in plasma are available, portable syringe-driven subcutaneous diamorphine infusion devices have proven clinical success. (Oliver, 1985; Wright and Callan, 1979; Jones and Hanks, 1986).

Oral

Bioavailability studies in animals with diamorphine using specific and sensitive methods for measuring the parent drug in plasma have not been reported.

Although much less potent when given orally, morphine and diamorphine have been widely used as an oral preparation for the treatment of chronic pain in man. From a study of 24-hour urine samples, collected after repeated administration of either morphine or diamorphine elixir for

Table 2.1 Physicochemical properties of diamorphine relevant to their pharmacokinetic behaviour.

PROPERTY	DIAMORPHINE HYDROCHLORIDE	6-O-ACETYL- MORPHINE	MORPHINE HYDROCHLORIDE	REFERENCE
pKa	7.83			Farmilo, et al. (1954).
	7.3(20°C)		8.0, 9.9 (20°C)	Pharmaceutical Codex (1979).
Solubility in water	1 in 1.6		1 in 24	Martindale (1982).
	500 mg/ml		60 mg/ml	Merk Index
Olive oil/ water partition coefficient	0.2		0.016	Oldendorf (1978).
n-heptane/ buffer pH 7.4 Log partition coefficient (23°C)	0.043 ±0.007	0.0012 ±0.00006	±0.00006 <0.00001	Umans and Inturrisi (1982).

3 days, 77% of diamorphine was excreted in urine as total morphine. A similar amount was excreted in the urine as total morphine after intravenous administration (Twycross et al., 1974). The similarity between these urinary recoveries indicates that when given orally in solution, diamorphine is well absorbed from the gastrointestinal tract in man. Although these results are indicative of extensive absorption, this does not equate to good bioavailability of diamorphine itself.

When measuring the plasma concentrations of non-conjugated morphine, Aherne et al., 1979, found similar results for diamorphine and morphine elixirs. However, it should be pointed out that the radio-immunoassay used was non-specific and could not differentiate between diamorphine, 6-O-acetylmorphine and morphine.

It was not until 1984 that a sufficiently sensitive high-pressure liquid chromatography method, specific for diamorphine in plasma, was developed (Inturrisi et al., 1984). Using this method it was shown that after oral administration of diamorphine, neither diamorphine nor 6-O-acetylmorphine were detected in blood. Furthermore the plasma levels of morphine following oral doses of diamorphine were approximately 20% lower than those for an equivalent dose of morphine.

'However, when differences in morphine dose due to administration of equal weights of diamorphine hydrochloride or morphine sulphate are taken into account, both opioid doses would be expected to yield approximately equivalent systemic concentrations of morphine.'

Urinary recovery of total morphine was not significantly different in addicts (Oberst, 1943) or ex-addicts (Yeh *et al.*, 1976), suggesting that the disposition of diamorphine is not altered after chronic use.

Intramuscular

After intramuscular administration peak plasma concentrations of diamorphine were seen at 10 minutes (Fig. 2.2) and by 30 minutes the plasma concentrations of the parent drug were not measurable (Inturrisi *et al*, 1984).

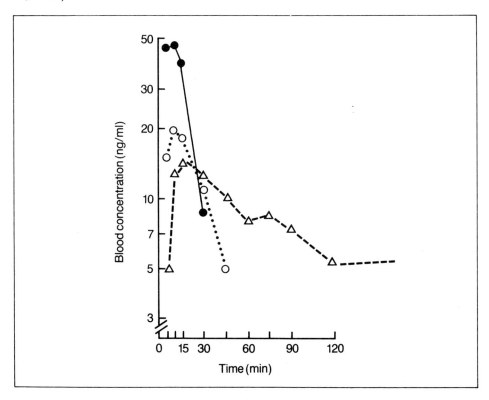

Fig. 2.2 Blood levels of diamorphine (closed circles) 6-O-acetylmorphine (open circles) and morphine (open triangles) after a single 4 mg intramuscular dose of diamorphine hydrochloride to a patient. (Produced, with permission, from the data of Inturrisi *et al.*, 1984.)

Inhalation

There have been no publications describing diamorphine bioavailability after inhalation other than one which compared urinary recoveries of total (free and conjugated) morphine after intravenous dosing and two modes of inhalation. The inhaled methods were 'chasing the dragon' (inhalation of fumes resulting from heating diamorphine and barbitone on a piece of aluminium foil), and 'ack-ack' (smoking cigarettes containing diamorphine powder). After intravenous, dragon-chasing and ack-ack modes of administration the 24-hour urinary recoveries of total morphine were 68%, 26% and 14% respectively. It was concluded that inhalation was not an effective route for administering diamorphine (Mo and Way, 1966).

Epidural and intrathecal

Intraspinal injections can be made epidurally, i.e., outside the dura mater or intrathecally, i.e., directly into the cerebrospinal fluid (CSF). Because of the diffusion barrier created by the dura mater, much higher doses of opioids are required when given epidurally compared to intrathecally.

The anatomical and physicochemical principles underlying the intrathecal and epidural administration of opiates have been reviewed by Cousins and Mather, 1984. Most studies of administration by these routes have compared and contrasted morphine with fentanyl, meperidine and methadone and, therefore, there have been few publications describing the pharmacokinetics of diamorphine after intrathecal or epidural dosing.

It is reasonable to accept that the pKa and lipid solubility of opioids can be used to explain differences in the onset, duration and intensity of analgesia after intrathecal and epidural dosing. Immediately after intrathecal injection of an opiate, very high concentrations of drug occur transiently within the CSF. These fall rapidly as a consequence of distribution away from the site of administration into the surrounding tissues, the spinal cord and blood vessels. Only relatively low concentrations of parent drug remain after a short time. If it is assumed that only nonionised lipophilic molecules can passively diffuse across membranes, the amount of drug able to transfer from the site of injection is related to its lipid solubility, the proportion of the drug present as the lipophilic, unionised form and the degree to which the drug binds to protein within the spinal cord and surrounding tissues. A highly ionised and relatively poorly lipid soluble opiate such as morphine will produce high concentrations of unbound drug in the CSF, whereas the more lipophilic, poorly ionised and highly protein-bound opioids like fentanyl, produce lower CSF concentrations of unbound drug. The ability to differentiate between the distribution of opiate drugs within the spinal cord is clearer when they are administered by the epidural route since another lipophilic membrane has

21

to be permeated. With epidural injections, morphine will only slowly leave the CSF due to poor lipid solubility, whereas the more lipophilic opiates, such as diamorphine and fentanyl, will readily cross these membranes resulting in rapid loss from the site of administration and rapid onset of effect within the spinal cord. With opioid drugs of limited lipid solubility the rate of penetration of the membrane will always determine the onset of the analgesic effect. Since the transfer of freely permeable drugs (e.g., fentanyl) is by passive diffusion, the time to onset of action can be shortened by increasing the dose. The influence of lipophilicity on the time to onset of action is clearly illustrated in Table 2.2.

The diffusion of an opioid from the site of administration into blood vessels within the spinal canal is also a major determinant of the rate of disappearance of the drug from the CSF or the epidural space into the systemic circulation. If the dose is sufficient, and significant amounts of drug are removed from the site of administration, some systemic analgesia may be produced. The rate of distribution away from the site of administration would also influence the rate of drug elimination. Therefore it is evident that both the times of onset and duration of spinal analgesia are a reflection of the degree of ionisation (pKa) and lipid solubility of opioid drugs. However, the affinity of the drug for the opioid receptor is also an important operating factor. It is to be expected that the duration of action of opioids such as buprenorphine which bind avidly to receptors, will be even longer, irrespective of their pharmacokinetic behaviour (Budd, 1981).

Table 2.2 Times of onset and duration of action of several opioid drugs, given epidurally. (Data taken from Naulty, 1986.)

DRUG	RELATIVE LIPID SOLUBILITY	DOSE (mg)	ONSET (min.)	DURATION (h)
Morphine	1	2.5–5	30–60	16–24
Methadone	82	5	15–20	6–8
Butorphanol	100	2–4	10–15	6–12
Diamorphine	200	5	9–15	6–12
Fentanyl	580	0.05–0.1	6–9	3–5
Lofentanil	1,035	0.001–0.005	2–5	8–10
Sufentanil	1,270	15–75	2–8	4–6

The clinical consequences of the ability of diamorphine to diffuse away from its epidural injection site more rapidly than morphine has been demonstrated in a study involving 27 patients undergoing thoracotomy (Phillips *et al.*, 1984). Concentrations of morphine in the plasma were consistently higher in patients receiving diamorphine than in a parallel group who received the same epidural dose of morphine (Fig. 2.3).

Detailed pharmacokinetic studies in which CSF concentrations of diamorphine and morphine were measured using a specific HPLC method were reported by Moore *et al.*, 1984. Diamorphine was removed from the CSF more rapidly than morphine (Fig. 2.4). The authors suggested that the short half-life of 6–8 minutes for diamorphine (14–360 minutes for morphine) was not due to diffusion across the dura mater which has low permeability to the drugs (Moore *et al.*, 1982) and in any event the concentrations (the main driving force of passive diffusion), were similar in both cases. The difference was thought to be due to the more rapid uptake of diamorphine into the spinal cord. Based only on the differences in half-life, the duration of action of diamorphine would be

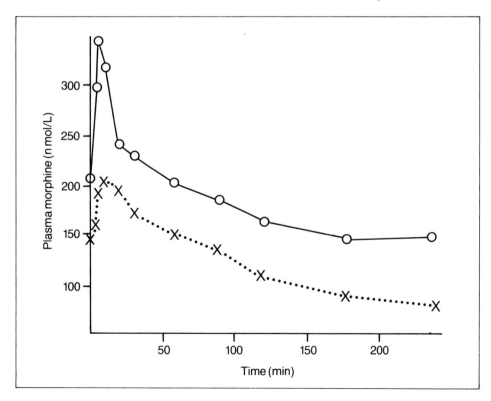

Fig. 2.3 Mean plasma concentrations of morphine after thoracic epidural injection of 2 mg morphine sulphate (crosses) or 2 mg diamorphine hydrochloride (open circles) to twenty-seven patients. (Reproduced, with permission, from Phillips *et al.*, 1984.)

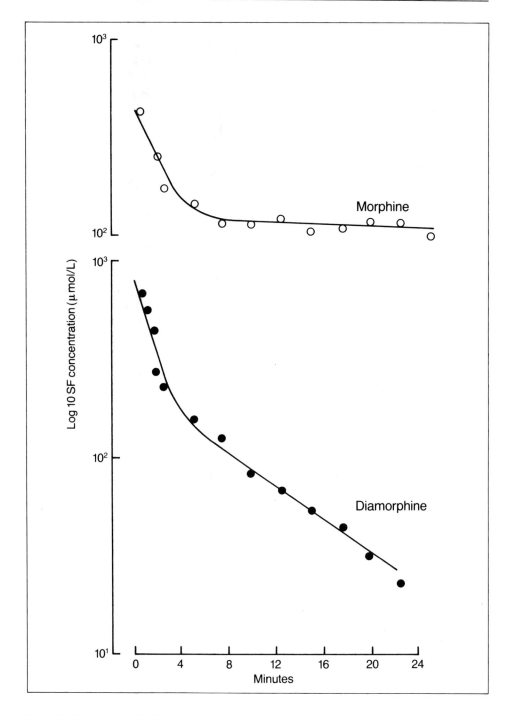

Fig. 2.4 Mean spinal fluid concentrations of morphine and diamorphine after intrathecal injection of 2.5 mg morphine sulphate or 2 mg diamorphine hydrochloride. The solid lines represent a computer-fitted biexponential equation. (Reproduced, with permission, from Moore *et al.*, 1984.)

expected to be much less than that for morphine. In clinical practice this is not so since diamorphine is metabolised within the spinal cord to morphine (Way et al., 1965). Furthermore, the detection limit for morphine in the spinal fluid studies (Moore et al., 1984) was 5 μmol/L and levels of 0.010 μmol/L have been shown to displace 50% of naloxone from opioid receptors (Pert and Snyder, 1973). Therefore, a significant analgesic effect due to metabolically-formed morphine could occur when spinal fluid levels were much less than the 5 μmol/L detectable by the relatively insensitive HPLC assay. These pharmacokinetic findings also indicate that rostral movement of diamorphine would be less than that for morphine and that this would lead to less late-onset respiratory depression with intrathecal diamorphine.

The relationships between lipophilicity and the CSF pharmacokinetics of these two opiates were further investigated by Moore and his colleagues in patients over a 6-hour period after intrathecal administration of morphine or diamorphine (Kotob et al., 1986). The mean elimination half-lives for morphine and diamorphine in spinal fluid were 73 and 43 minutes respectively. Both opiates were cleared from spinal fluid at approximately 0.6–0.7 ml/min. The plasma concentration of the 2 drugs were very different (Fig. 2.5) and indicative of rapid removal of diamorphine by diffusion (presumably into the blood supplying the spinal cord) and subsequent rapid deacetylation to morphine.

In patients undergoing lumbar laminectomy, and given extradural doses of either morphine or diamorphine, the peak plasma concentration occurred significantly earlier after diamorphine (about 5 minutes) than after morphine (about 10 minutes), and was also significantly higher after diamorphine (Watson et al., 1984). Using estimates of the elimination- and absorption-rate constants, the authors were able to estimate that the fraction of epidural diamorphine which crossed the dura was 55% of the respective value for morphine.

Intravenous

The pharmacokinetic properties of diamorphine can only be obtained from those studies where specific and sensitive methods exist for the detection and measurement of the drug in plasma and other biological fluids. In the majority of the publications describing diamorphine disposition in animals and man, the methods have either not been sufficiently sensitive (Elliot et al., 1971) or specific (Aherne et al., 1975) to allow a description of diamorphine pharmacokinetics. Determination of diamorphine in blood or plasma is further complicated by the spontaneous ex vivo metabolism to 6-O-acetylmorphine (Nakamura et al., 1975; Smith and

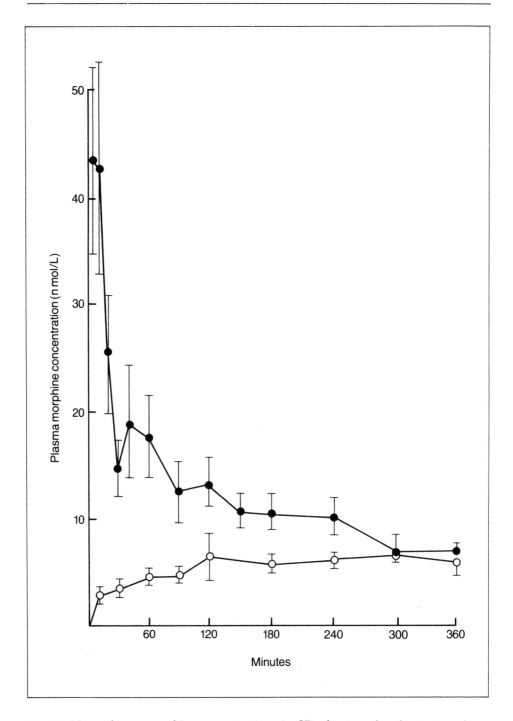

Fig. 2.5 Mean plasma morphine concentrations (± SE) after intrathecal injection of 1 mg of morphine sulphate (open circles) or 1 mg of anhydrous diamorphine hydrochloride (closed circles) to patients. (Reproduced, with permission, from Kotob *et al.*, 1986.)

Cole, 1976; Lockeridge et al., 1980). Inhibition of diamorphine hydrolysis to 6-O-acetylmorphine was reported by Garrett and Gurkan, 1979, who used this approach, coupled with thin layer chromatography, to define the pharmacokinetic behaviour of unchanged drug, 6-O-acetylmorphine, morphine and their various glucuronide conjugates in a dog after intravenous administration of diamorphine (Garrett and Gurkan, 1980). Plasma profiles of diamorphine were described using a triexponential equation which implies that the rapid decrease in concentration was due to extensive distribution into the tissues plus concomitant metabolic elimination. The total body clearance was six times higher than hepatic blood flow in the dog and suggests considerable extrahepatic elimination since less than 2% of the dose was renally cleared. The notion of extensive distribution into the tissues is also supported by a volume of distribution of about 350 l, some 15–20 times body weight, and suggests that the lipophilic drug is taken up into lipid-containing tissues such as the CNS and body fat. The total clearance and volume of distribution of morphine in this study were slightly less than the corresponding values for diamorphine. This study also showed that diamorphine was simultaneously metabolised to equal amounts of 6-O-acetylmorphine and morphine.

Hepatic extraction studies in an isolated perfused rabbit liver preparation showed quite clearly that morphine was less avidly cleared by rabbit liver than was diamorphine (Kreek et al., 1978).

Extrahepatic elimination was also observed in man by Inturrisi et al., 1984, who found that after bolus intravenous or intramuscular injections of diamorphine (4–16 mg), blood concentrations of the parent drug declined rapidly during the first 10 minutes, due to metabolic clearance in the blood and various body organs, plus local degradation. During continuous intravenous infusion to patients with chronic pain, the parent drug and its metabolite 6-O-acetylmorphine quickly achieved an apparent steady-state blood concentration consistent with the short half-life of diamorphine. Doubling the infusion rate resulted in an approximate doubling of the apparent steady-state blood concentrations and a constant blood clearance of approximately 2100 ml/min (3.1 ml/min/kg).

The limited results from this study demonstrate that for infusion rates of up to 333 mg/min the pharmacokinetics of diamorphine remain independent of dose.

In the absence of any significant contribution of renal elimination to diamorphine clearance, the oral bioavailability (F) is related to the hepatic extraction ratio (ER_H) thus:

$$F = 1 - ER_H$$

Clearance through the liver (Cl_H) is dependent upon hepatic blood-flow (Q_H) and hepatic extraction ratio (ER_H) thus:

$$Cl_H = Q_H \times ER_H$$

The data from man and dog show that the total blood clearance of diamorphine is greater than liver blood flow (i.e., $Cl_H >> Q_H$) consequently the hepatic extraction ratio approximates to unity. Therefore it could be predicted from intravenous studies that the oral bioavailability of diamorphine is very low. This is borne out by the evidence that no diamorphine was detected in plasma after oral dosing (Inturrisi *et al.*, 1984).

The pharmacokinetic properties of diamorphine are entirely consistent with those for a drug of abuse and physical dependence. Enhanced self-administration is associated with rapid absorption (availability of morphine), rapid entry into specific brain regions, low protein binding, short half-life and high clearance (Busto and Sellers, 1986). These are all true for diamorphine, especially when given by intravenous injection.

The application of a specific method for measuring diamorphine in plasma has clearly shown that in those earlier studies, where a pharmacological effect was used to assess absorption, this was more than likely due to the formation of pharmacologically-active metabolites, and not to the systemic availability of parent drug. In man the oral bioavailability of diamorphine is negligible and, after intramuscular dosing, the plasma levels are low and fall to undetectable levels within 30 minutes. Direct administration of diamorphine into the epidural and intrathecal spaces produces CSF concentrations, far greater than those seen after intravenous injection.

Distribution

Very few quantitative studies have been carried out on the distribution of diamorphine, probably due to the instability of the drug in the majority of body fluids and tissues.

Blood–brain penetration

Tissue concentrations of ^{11}C-labelled morphine or diamorphine after intravenous injection in rats showed that 40% of the radioactivity was seen in the small intestine, with smaller amounts in the liver and kidney, but little activity was detected in the brain. Although much less diamorphine was detected in the brain, it was still three times the equivalent amount of morphine (Kloster *et al.*, 1979). A similar study in Rhesus monkeys, using positron-emission tomography, which allows for the measurement of radioactivity in discrete organs while maintaining normal physiology, indicated that the maximum normalised uptake for diamorphine and ^{11}C-morphine in the brain was 4.6 and 0.2 respectively. Maximum radioactivity in the brain was reached 35–45 minutes after administration of ^{11}C-morphine and the half-life was greater than 2 hours, whereas ^{11}C-diamorphine reached peak radioactivity levels earlier and its half-life was considerably shorter (Hartvig *et al.*, 1984).

The ability for rapid uptake of diamorphine into the brain was also demonstrated by measuring the amount of radiolabelled diamorphine and other opiates taken up by the brain during a single passage, after injection into the rat carotid artery. While levels of morphine were undetectable, $68 \pm 6\%$ of the radiolabelled diamorphine was taken up into the brain (Oldendorf *et al.*, 1972). Hence, in comparison with other opiates, diamorphine equilibrates rapidly across the blood-brain barrier (Fig. 2.6). The differences in brain uptake between these opiates has been attributed to a

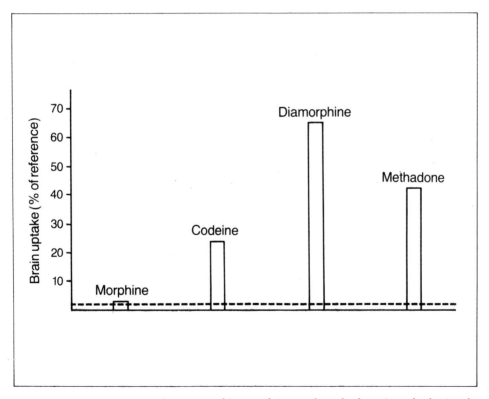

Fig. 2.6 Uptake of diamorphine, morphine, codeine and methadone into the brain of a rat after administration into the carotid artery. (Reproduced, with permission, from Oldendorf *et al.*, 1972.)

relationship involving their degree of ionisation at plasma pH and the oil/water partition coefficient (Oldendorf, 1974). The general dependence of brain uptake and these physicochemical parameters is shown in Fig. 2.7.

Distribution in man

Studies on the distribution of diamorphine and its metabolites in man, have been limited to detection and measurement in various body fluids and tissues including saliva, spinal fluid, foetal blood, blood within the umbilical cord and an assortment of post-mortem tissue samples.

The use of saliva and plasma concentrations in detecting high-dose chronic diamorphine abuse was evaluated in healthy volunteers after the administration of single intravenous doses (2.5, 5 and 10 mg per 70 kg). Low doses were not detectable in either the plasma or saliva but with the higher doses detection of opiate was possible for 2–4 hours in the plasma and 1–2 hours in saliva. These times increased during chronic morphine administration to 6 hours and 3–4 hours respectively. The plasma and saliva samples may be of use in detecting chronic drug abuse (Gorodetzky and Kullberg, 1974).

Post-mortem distribution of morphine in diamorphine addicts is found to be extremely variable but certain features are apparent. Bound morphine in the liver accounts for 70% of the total concentration in that organ which is usually greater than in the kidney. Morphine may or may not be found in blood at post-mortem examination (Robinson and Williams 1971).

Placental transfer

Several studies have demonstrated that diamorphine and its metabolites very rapidly cross the mammalian placenta into the foetal circulation, and may cause respiratory depression and other problems (Finnegan, 1976; Cravey and Reed, 1981). Apart from its teratogenic effects in causing growth retardation (Finnegan, 1981), neonates born to diamorphine-addicted mothers often experience postpartum withdrawal syndromes (Klenka, 1986).

In obstetric patients receiving intramuscular diamorphine (10 mg), the mean umbilical cord/maternal plasma ratio of 'morphine equivalents' at delivery was 1.59 ± 0.84, determined by radioimmunoassay. During the first 24 hours following birth, the concentration of 'morphine equivalents' in neonatal plasma declined from a mean of 17.2 ng/ml at 4 hours to 3.2 ng/ml at 24 hours. There were no obvious dose-related differences (Freeman *et al.*, 1982), and the authors concluded that obstetric use of diamorphine may be advantageous over that of pethidine since foetal concentrations decline rapidly.

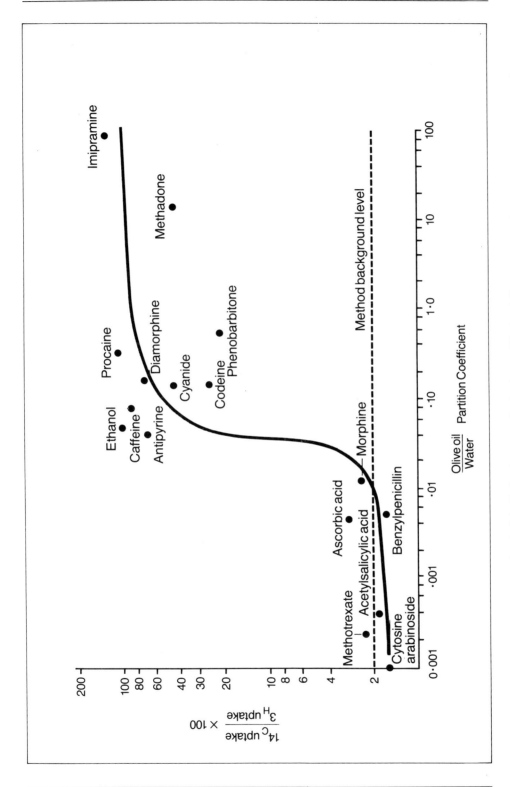

Fig. 2.7 A plot of percent clearance of radiolabelled substances by brain capilliaries following carotid artery injection against the respective olive oil/water partition coefficient for a number of drugs. (Reproduced, with permission, from Oldendorf, 1974.)

31

The data of Freeman *et al.*, 1982, show an estimated half-life for 'morphine equivalents' in the neonate of about 5 hours. Corresponding half-life estimates for the maternal plasma are approximately twofold lower at 2.7 hours. Since foetal metabolic capacity is considerably under-developed in the immediate post-natal period, it can be expected that elimination of opiate materials from the neonate would be less than that for the mother.

Protein binding

The binding properties of diamorphine and its metabolites to proteins or red blood cells in human blood were studied *in vitro* and neither diamorphine nor morphine exhibited significant binding with physiological levels of various proteins (Cohn *et al.*, 1974). In contrast, Comparini *et al.*, 1985, using proton spin-lattice relaxation rates, suggested that diamorphine did undergo some binding interaction with receptor sites located in whole human blood or plasma and tentatively suggested that fibrinogen was the responsible protein molecule. Using a sufficiently sensitive method for measuring ^{14}C-diamorphine in plasma, Garrett and Gurkan, 1979, were able to show that, contrary to the findings of Cohn *et al.*, diamorphine was approximately 40% bound to plasma proteins and was not taken up into the erythrocytes.

One important aspect of binding to macromolecules is that of binding to the opiate receptor in the brain. The unsubstituted phenolic hydroxyl group at C3 of the morphine nucleus (Fig. 2.8) has been shown to be required for *in vitro* opiate receptor binding and is presumably important for the *in vivo* analgesic activity. The relative opiate receptor binding affinities of diamorphine, 6-O-acetylmorphine and morphine were assessed in the rat brain by measuring their ability to displace ^{3}H-naltrexone from opiate binding sites. Diamorphine was found not to bind to these receptors but 6-O-acetylmorphine and morphine did, readily. This infers that diamorphine lacks intrinsic opiate activity but acts as a highly lipophilic prodrug that serves to determine the distribution of its active metabolites to these receptors (Inturrisi *et al.*, 1983).

Metabolism

Studies by Kemp and Way, 1954, indicated that the metabolism of diamorphine occurred in homogenates of brain, kidney, liver, and in blood from humans, dogs, rats, rabbits and mice. Liver tissue was the most active and brain tissue was the least active.

It appeared from these *in vitro* studies that all the tissues examined

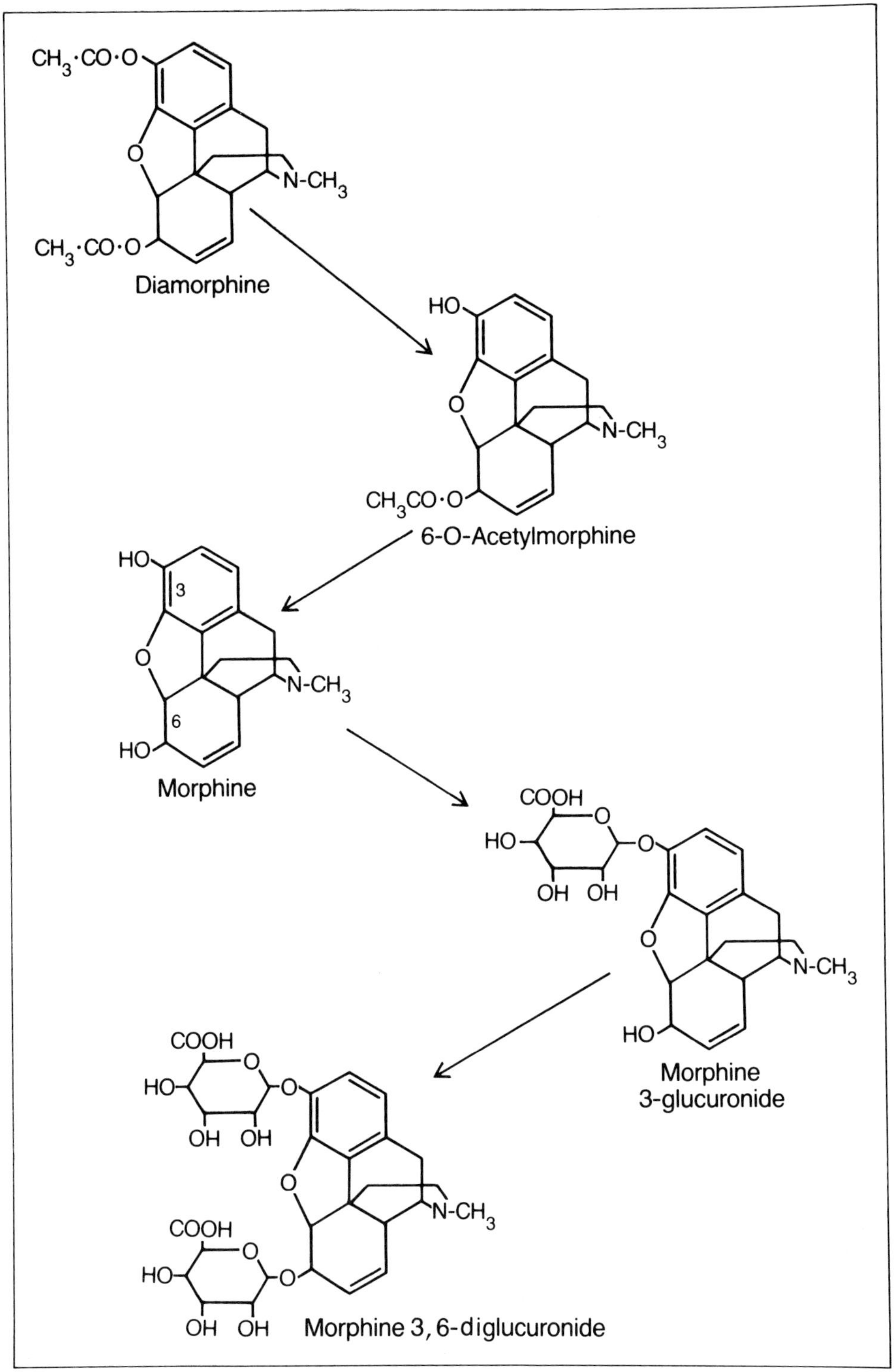

Fig. 2.8 Pathways of diamorphine metabolism.

showed considerable but varying degrees of ability to metabolise diamorphine to 6-O-acetylmorphine and morphine.

In serum, diamorphine was rapidly deacetylated to 6-0-monoacetylmorphine which was stable for up to 7 hours. However, only a small amount of morphine was formed, whereas, when diamorphine was incubated with whole blood, morphine was detected in greater amounts. In both serum and whole blood, the levels of 6-O-acetylmorphine remained relatively large. Diamorphine hydrolysis therefore occurred much more rapidly in whole blood than in serum with half-lives of 9 and 22 minutes respectively (Nakamura *et al.*, 1975).

Hence, there is well-documented evidence that diamorphine is rapidly hydrolysed in the body to 6-O-acetylmorphine and then more slowly to morphine, both of which have pharmacological activity. 6-O-acetylmorphine has been shown to enter the central nervous system and brain very rapidly, where it achieves high concentrations and then is more slowly metabolised to morphine which, in contrast, is far less lipophilic and so cannot easily enter or leave the central nervous system (Way *et al.*, 1960). This group of workers postulated that morphine is the major pharmacologically active agent and that diamorphine and 6-O-acetylmorphine are precursors which facilitate the entry of morphine into the brain (Way *et al.*, 1965). This greater ability of diamorphine and 6-O-acetylmorphine to penetrate the blood-brain barrier serves to explain the higher potency of diamorphine compared to morphine and its more rapid onset of action. As diamorphine and 6-O-acetylmorphine are equipotent, diamorphine acts principally as its metabolites (Lockridge *et al.*, 1980).

The identity of the enzyme or enzymes responsible for the metabolism of diamorphine has not been clearly established (Williams, 1985). Most studies have been conducted in blood which is known to hydrolyse diamorphine very quickly. That its metabolism is enzyme-mediated was established by Nakamura and Ukita, 1967. When large amounts of diamorphine were measured in enzyme-deactivated blood, it was shown that diamorphine does not spontaneously hydrolyse to 6-O-acetylmorphine. Early workers concluded that serum cholinesterase was not responsible (Wright, 1942) but that tributyrinase was involved (Ellis, 1948). Using blood from healthy volunteers, Smith and Cole, 1976, determined that plasma arylesterase was responsible for deacetylating 30–35% diamorphine to 6-O-acetylmorphine and that the remaining hydrolysis occurred in association with red blood cells. However, Lockridge *et al.*, 1980, presented data to suggest that cholinesterase was responsible for diamorphine hydrolysis, but could not identify the enzyme that hydrolyses 6-O-acetylmorphine to morphine. The rate of diamorphine hydrolysis is sufficiently fast to claim that blood is the major site of 6-O-acetylmorphine production after intravenous administration.

The involvement of serum cholinesterase in the hydrolysis of diamorphine was supported by Owen and Nakatsu, 1983, but they actually identified four distinct enzymes capable of diamorphine hydrolysis in human blood fractions. They confirmed that the plasma enzyme was cholinesterase but that three separate enzymes found were responsible for nearly 70% of the hydrolysis in blood.

The importance of central and peripheral esterases in various tissues was examined in mice using tri-ortho-tolyl (TOTP) to selectively inhibit peripheral cholinesterase and carboxylesterase activity without inhibiting brain activity, and paraoxon to inhibit in vitro brain activity. This study confirmed that the greater potency of diamorphine over morphine is due to pharmacokinetic factors rather than enhanced intrinsic pharmacological activity since it is considerably less avidly taken up by the opiate-binding sites. The authors suggested that central esterases may activate diamorphine near the site of action while peripheral esterases participate in its metabolism and excretion (Gianutsos et al., 1986).

In summary, diamorphine is rapidly deacetylated in the body to 6-O-acetylmorphine and then to morphine which is conjugated with glucuronic acid (Fig. 2.8). The pharmacologic activity of 6-O-acetylmorphine is equipotent to diamorphine and it has been suggested that diamorphine acts principally as 6-O-acetylmorphine (Boerner et al., 1975; Inturrisi et al., 1983).

Excretion

When diamorphine was administered as a constant intravenous infusion in humans, at a rate of 10 mg/hour, 43.6% of the administered doses was recoverable as morphine, 0.13% as diamorphine, and 1.3% as 6-O-acetylmorphine in the urine collected over 40 hours (Elliot et al., 1971). Morphine is excreted partly as free substance and partly conjugated as the glucuronide. Total morphine (free and conjugated) excretion in the urine after 10 mg/70 kg diamorphine hydrochloride in 10 subjects was $74.94 \pm 4.4\%$, but only $7.82 \pm 0.89\%$ of this amount was as free substance; over 65% of the recoverable amount was collected within 8 hours of administration (Yeh et al., 1976). Diamorphine is excreted mainly as conjugated morphine in the urine (50–60%) (Garrett and Gurkan 1980; Yeh et al., 1977; Garrett and Gurkan 1979), with the ratio of free to conjugated, 1:9.1 (Boerner et al., 1975).

Pharmacokinetic interactions between diamorphine and other drugs

Pharmacokinetic drug interactions occur when one drug alters the absorption, distribution or elimination of another. This may result in an alteration in the clinical response, depending upon the degree of the interaction and the relationship between drug concentration and response. The severity of the interaction may warrant dosage adjustments and, equally, care must be taken when stopping treatment with one drug which is known to interact with another. Comprehensive reviews on the pharmacokinetic basis of drug interactions have been presented elsewhere (Kristensen, 1983).

An interaction with the absorption of a drug may be a physicochemical phenomenon (i.e., raised solubility/dissolution or altered stability, etc.), or may arise from an alteration in one of the physiological processes involved in absorption (e.g., gastrointestinal motility, mesenteric blood flow, etc.).

Diamorphine, like other narcotic analgesics has marked effects on gastrointestinal smooth muscle in that it delays gastric transit and inhibits gastric emptying (Jaffe and Martin, 1985). Intramuscular doses of diamorphine (10 mg) dramatically reduced the rate of paracetamol absorption in volunteers. This was attributed to considerable delay (approximately 1.5 h) in the transit of paracetamol from the stomach into the small intestine (Nimmo *et al.*, 1975a). A similar effect on paracetamol absorption was seen in patients, receiving intramuscular doses of diamorphine following hysterectomy. Those patients who were given epidural local anaesthetic showed only a moderate (non-significant) delay in paracetamol absorption (Nimmo *et al.*, 1978). The ability of diamorphine to alter gastric emptying was further studied in women during labour. Paracetamol absorption (i.e., gastric emptying) was normal during labour in women who had not received narcotic analgesics, whereas its absorption was severely delayed in those patients receiving diamorphine, pethidine or pentazocine. These effects were not reversed by metaclopramide (Nimmo *et al.*, 1975b). It has been suggested by the same group that the absorption of oral antiarrhythmics is also reduced when given with narcotic analgesics (Prescott, 1980).

Interactions between opioid drugs and ethanol have been extensively studied in animals and man using methadone as the model drug. This work has been reviewed by Kreek, 1984, who concludes, that in the addicted diamorphine-user the 'need' for the drug may be exacerbated by concomitant alcohol abuse. Ethanol-induced metabolic activity has been implicated in the complex situation arising in those diamorphine addicts who are also chronic alcohol-drinkers, since ethanol-induced cirrhosis is a common feature of their alcoholism.

In summary, the available evidence suggests that intramuscular doses of diamorphine delays gastric emptying and thereby may influence the absorption of other drugs. The clinical significance of this was raised in relation to the case of narcotic analgesics in women during labour, but other (significant) clinical manifestations of this potential have been reported.

There is no evidence to suggest that diamorphine interacts with the distribution or elimination of other drugs.

Studies in the rat have shown that the deacetylation of diamorphine in the liver is significantly enhanced in those animals pretreated with phenobarbitone (Cramer *et al.*, 1975) or high dose steroids (Cramer *et al.*, 1974). There have not been any publications describing changes in diamorphine pharmacokinetics in the presence of other drugs in man.

Detection and measurement of diamorphine and morphine in biological fluids

A description of the pharmacokinetic characteristics of a drug relies upon the measurement of drug concentrations in plasma (or urine) using a specific and sufficiently sensitive analytical procedure. When non-specific analytical procedures are used, the methods employed in describing plasma concentration versus time profiles and deriving pharmacokinetic characteristics become invalid. Analytical sensitivity is required to ensure that plasma drug concentrations are monitored over a sufficiently long time period to warrant pharmacokinetic description.

There are many publications describing numerous methods for the detection and quantification of diamorphine and morphine in plasma and urine. The key review articles and original reports of the more commonly used methods are given in Table 2.3 along with brief comments. The radioimmunoassay methods also detects 6-O-acetylmorphine and morphine and therefore is non-specific yet sensitive. The methods of choice for pharmacokinetic studies are HPLC and gas chromatography.

Conclusion

Diamorphine is rapidly metabolised to 6-O-acetylmorphine and morphine, both of which possess considerable pharmacological activity. The relative contribution of diamorphine 6-O-acetylmorphine and morphine

Table 2.3 Methods for the measurement of diamorphine in plasma and urine.

ANALYTICAL METHOD	COMMENTS	REFERENCE
Plasma		
Radioimmunoassay	Non specific – also measures morphine and 6-O-acetylmorphine	Gorodetzky and Kullberg, 1974 Castro and Mittleman, 1978 Harwood, 1974 Aherne *et al.*, 1975
Gas chromatography	Specific	Smith and Cole 1975
Mass fragmentography	Specific, expensive	Cole *et al.*, 1977 Ebbighausen *et al.*, 1974
High performance liquid chromatography (HPLC)	Specific, inexpensive	Umans *et al.*, 1982 Garrett and Gurkan, 1979
Urine		
Thin-layer chromatography	Identification of metabolites only	Yeh *et al.*, 1977
Various	Review article	Gorodetzky *et al.*, 1974

to the overall analgesic response is largely determined by differences in their physicochemical and pharmacokinetic properties. This is particularly true for their permeability across the blood-brain barrier into the CSF and disposition after either intrathecal or epidural dosing. Detailed pharmacokinetic studies with vascular and extravascular doses of diamorphine have not been carried out because specific assay methods with sufficient sensitivity have not been employed.

References

Aherne, G. W., Marks, V., Morris, B. A., Piall, E. M., Robinson, J. D. and Twycross, R. G., (1975), 'The measurement of serum morphine levels by radioimmunoassay following oral administration of diamorphine or morphine', *British Journal of Pharmacology*, **54**, 228.

Aherne, G. W., Piall, E. M. and Twycross, R. G., (1979), 'Serum morphine concentration after oral administration of diamorphine hydrochloride and morphine sulphate', *British Journal of Clinical Pharmacology*, **8**, 577.

Boerner, U., Abbott, S. and Roe, R. L., (1975), 'The metabolism of morphine and heroin in man', *Drug Metabolism Reviews*, **4**, 39.

Budd, K., (1981), 'High dose buprenorphine for post-operative analgesia', *Anaesthesia*, **36**, 900.

Busto, U. and Sellers, E. M., (1986), 'Pharmacokinetic determinants of drug abuse and dependence', *Clinical Pharmacokinetics*, **11**, 144.

Camparini, I. B., Gaggelli, E., Marchettini, N. and Valensin, G., (1985), 'Binding features of diacetylmorphine (heroin) in whole blood and in blood fractions', *Biophysical Journal*, **48**, 247.

Castro, A. and Mittleman, R., (1978), 'Determination of drugs of abuse in body fluids by radioimmunoassay', *Clinical Biochemistry*, **11**, 103.

Cohn, G. L., Cramer, J. A., McBride, W., Brown, R. C. and Kleber, H. D., (1974), 'Heroin and morphine binding with human serum proteins and red blood cells', *Proceedings of the Society of Experimental Biological Medicine*, **147**, 664.

Cole, W. J., Parkhouse, J. and Yousef, Y. Y., (1977), 'Application of the extractive alkylation technique to the pentafluorobenzylation of morphine and surrogates with special reference to the quantitative determination of plasma morphine levels using mass fragmentography', *Journal of Chromatography*, **136**, 409.

Cousins, M. J. and Mather, L. E., (1984), 'Intrathecal and epidural administration of opioids', *Anaesthesiology*, **61**, 276.

Cramer, J., Cohn, G. and Kleber, H., (1974), 'Effect of steroids on heroin metabolism in the rat', *Federation Proceedings*, **33**, 478.

Cramer, J., Cohn, G. and Meggs, L., (1975), 'Effect of phenobarbitone on heroin metabolism in the rat', *Federation Proceedings*, **34**, 3,362.

Cravey, R. H. and Reed, D., (1981), 'Placental transfer of narcotic analgesics in man', *Clinical Toxicology*, **18**, 911.

Dutt, M. C., (1984), 'Laboratory diagnosis of opiate drugs', *Annals of the Academy of Medicine, Singapore*, **13**, 53.

Ebbighausen, W. O. R., Mowat, J. H., Stearns, H. and Vestergaard, P., (1974), 'Mass fragmentography of morphine and 6-0-monoacetylmorphine in blood with a stable isotope internal standard', *Biomedical Mass Spectrometry*, **1**, 305.

Elliot, H. W., Parker, K. D., Wright, J. A. and Nomof, N., (1971), 'Actions and metabolism of heroin administered by continuous intravenous infusion to man', *Clinical Pharmacology and Therapeutics*, **12**, 806.

Farmilo, C. G., Oestreicher, P. M. and Levi, L., (1954), 'The physical methods for the identification of narcotics', *Bulletin of Narcotics*, **6**, 7.

Finnegan, L. P., (1976), 'Clinical effects of pharmacologic agents on pregnancy, the foetus and the neonate', *Annals of New York Academy of Science*, **281**, 74.

Finnegan, L. P., (1981), 'The effects of narcotics and alcohol on pregnancy and the newborn', *Annals of New York Academy of Science*, **362**, 136.

Freeman, R. M., Moreland, T. A. and Blair, A. W., (1982), 'Diamorphine, the obstetric analgesic: a neurobehavioural and pharmacokinetic study in the neonate', *Journal of Obstetrics and Gynaecology*, **3**, 102.

Garrett, E. R. and Gurkan, T., (1979), 'Pharmacokinetics of morphine and its surrogates II. Methods of separation and stabilised heroin and its metabolites from hydrolysing biological fluids and applications to protein binding and red blood cell partition studies', *Journal of Pharmacological Sciences*, **68**, 26.

Garrett, E. R. and Gurkan, T., (1980), 'Pharmacokinetics of morphine and its surrogates IV. Pharmacokinetics of heroin and its derived metabolites in dogs', *Journal of Pharmacological Sciences*, **69**, 1,116.

Gianutsos, G., Cohen, S. D., Carlson, G., Heyman, R., Salva, P., Morrow, G. and Hite, G. J., (1986), 'Alteration of invivo and invitro effects of heroin by esterase inhibition', *Toxicology and Applied Pharmacology*, **82**, 14.

Gorodetzky, C. W., Angel, C. R., Beach, D. J., Catlin, D. H. and Yeh, S-Y., (1974), 'Validity of screening methods for drugs of abuse in biological fluids. I. Heroin in urine', *Clinical Pharmacology and Therapeutics*, **15**, 461.

Gorodetzky, C. W. and Kullberg, M. P., (1974), 'Validity of screening methods for drugs of abuse in biological fluids. II. Heroin in plasma and saliva', *Clinical Pharmacology and Therapeutics*, **15**, 579.

Gough, T. A. and Baker, P. B., (1983), 'Identification of major drugs of abuse using chromatography: An update', *Journal of Chromatographic Science*, **21**, 145.

Hartvig, P., Bergstrom, K., Lindberg, B., Lundberg, P. O., Lundqvist, H., Langstrom, B., Svard, H. and Rane, A., (1984), 'Kinetics of ^{11}C-labelled opiates in the brain of rhesus monkeys', *Journals of Pharmacology and Experimental Therapeutics*, **230**, 250.

Harwood, C. T., (1974), 'Radioimmunoassay: its application to drugs of abuse', *Pharmacology*, **11**, 52.

Hays, S. E., Grady, L. T. and Kruegal, A. V., (1973), 'Purity profiles for heroin, morphine and morphine hydrochloride', *Journal of Pharmacological Sciences*, **62**, 1,509.

Inturrisi, C. E., Schultz, M., Shin, S., Umans, J. G., Angel, L. and Simon, E. J., (1983), 'Evidence from opiate binding studies that heroin acts through its metabolites', *Life Sciences*, **33** (suppl. I), 773.

Inturrisi, C. E., Max, M. B., Foley, K. M., Schultz, M., Shin, S-U. and Houde, R. W., (1984), 'The pharmacokinetics of heroin in patients with chronic pain', *New England Journal of Medicine*, **310**, 1,213.

Jaffe, J. H. and Martin, W. R., (1985), 'Opioid analgesics and antagonists' in *The Pharmacological Basis of Therapeutics*. Gillman, A. G., Goodman, L. S., Rall, T. W. and Murad, F. (eds), (London, Collier Macmillan, 7th edition, p. 491).

Jones, V. A. and Hanks, G. W., (1986), 'New portable infusion pump for prolonged subcutaneous administration of opioid analgesics in patients with advanced cancer', *British Medical Journal*, **292**, 1,496.

Klenka, H. M., (1986), 'Babies born in a district general hospital to mothers taking heroin', *British Medical Journal*, **293**, 745.

Kloster, G., Roder, E. and Machulla, H-J., (1979), 'Synthesis, chromatography and tissue distribution of methyl-^{11}C-morphine and methyl-^{11}C-heroin', *Journal of Labelled Compounds and Radiopharmacy*, **16**, 441.

Kotob, H. I. M., Hand, C. W., Moore, R. A., Evans, P. J. D., Wells, J., Rubin, A. P. and McQuay, H. J., (1986), 'Intrathecal morphine and heroin in humans: six hour drug levels in spinal fluid and plasma', *Anesthesia and Analgesia*, **65**, 718.

Kreek, M. J., (1984), 'Opioid interactions with alcohol', *Advances in Alcohol and Substance Abuse*, **3**, 35.

Kreek, M. J., Oratz, M. and Rothschild, M. A. (1978), 'Hepatic extraction of long and short acting narcotics in the isolated perfused rabbit liver', *Gastroenterology*, **75**, 88.

Kristensen, M. B., (1983), 'Drug interactions and clinical pharmacokinetics' in *Handbook of Clinical Pharmacokinetics*, Gibaldi, M. and Prescott, L. F. (eds), (Balgowlah, Australia, ADIS Health Science Press, p. 242).

Lockeridge, O., Mottershaw-Jackson, N., Eckerson, H. W. and Ladu, B. N., (1980), 'Hydrolysis of diacetylmorphine (heroin) by human serum cholinesterase', *Journal of Pharmacology and Experimental Therapeutics*, **215**, 1.

Martindale, (1982), *The Extra Pharmacopoeia*, Reynolds, J. E. F. (ed), (London, The Pharmaceutical Press, 28th edition).

Misra, A. L., (1978), 'Metabolism of opiates' in *Factors Affecting the Action of Narcotics*, Adler, Manara and Samanin (eds), (New York, Raven Press).

Mo, B. P-N. and Way, E. L., (1966), 'An assessment of inhalation as a mode of administration of heroin by addicts', *Journal of Pharmacology and Experimental Therapeutics*, **154**, 142.

Moore, R. A., Bullingham, R. E. S., McQuay, H. J., Hand, C. W., Aspel, J. B., Allen, M. C. and Thomas, D., (1982), 'Dural permeability to narcotics; in vitro determination and application to extradural administration', *British Journal of Anaesthesia*, **54**, 1,117.

Moore, R. A., Bullingham, R., McQuay, H., Allen, M., Baldwin, D. and Cole, A., (1984), 'Spinal fluid kinetics of morphine and heroin', *Clinical Pharmacology and Therapeutics*, **35**, 40.

Nakamura, G. R., Thornton, J. and Noguchi, T. T., (1975), 'Kinetics of heroin deacetylation in aqueous alkaline solution and in human serum and whole blood', *Journal of Chromatography*, **110**, 81.

Nakamura, G. R. and Ukita, T., (1967), 'Paper chromatography study of in vitro and in vivo hydrolysis of heroin in blood', *Journal of Pharmacological Science*, **56**, 294.

Naulty, J. S., (1986), 'Intraspinal narcotics', *Clinics in Anaesthesiology*, **4**, 145.

Nimmo, W. S., Heading, R. C., Wilson, J., Tothill, P. and Prescott, L. F., (1975), 'Inhibition of gastric emptying and drug absorption by narcotic analgesics', *British Journal of Clinical Pharmacology*, **2**, 509.

Nimmo, W. S., Wilson, J. and Prescott, L. F., (1975), 'Narcotic analgesics and delayed gastric emptying in labour', *Lancet*, **i**, 890.

Nimmo, W. S., Littlewood, D. G., Scott, D. B. and Prescott, L. F., (1978), 'Gastric emptying following hysterectomy with extradural anaesthesia', *British Journal of Anaesthesia*, **50**, 559.

Oberst, F. W., (1943), 'Studies on the fate of heroin', *Journal of Pharmacology and Experimental Therapeutics*, **79**, 266.

Oldendorf, W. H., (1974), 'Blood-brain permeability to drugs', *Annual Review of Pharmacology*, **14**, 239.

Oldendorf, W. H., (1978), 'Factors affecting passage of opiates through the blood brain barrier' in *Factors Affecting the Action of Narcotics*, Adler, Manara and Samanin (eds), (New York, Raven Press, p. 221).

Oldendorf, W. H., Hyman, S., Braun, L. and Oldendorf, S. Z., (1972), 'Blood-brain barrier: penetration of morphine, codeine, heroin and methadone after carotid injection', *Science*, **178**, 984.

Oliver, D. J., (1985), 'The use of the syringe driver in terminal care', *British Journal of Clinical Pharmacology*, **20**, 515.

Owen, J. A., and Nakatsu, K., (1982), 'Diacetylmorphine (heroin) hydrolases in human blood', *Canadian Journal of Physiology and Pharmacology*, **61**, 870.

Pert, C. B., and Snyder, S. H., (1973), 'Properties of opiate receptor binding in rat brain', *Proceedings of the National Academy of Sciences*, **70**, 2,243.

Phillips, D. M., Moore, R. A., Bullingham, R. E. S., Allen, M. C., Baldwin, D., Fisher, A., Lloyd, J. W. and McQuay, H. J., (1984), 'Plasma morphine concentrations and clinical effects after thoracic extradural morphine or diamorphine', *British Journal of Anaesthesia*, **56**, 829.

Robinson, A. E. and Williams, F. M., (1971), 'Post-mortem distribution of morphine in heroin addicts', *Medicine, Science and the Law*, **11**, 135.

Sawynok, J., (1986), 'The therapeutic use of heroin: a review of the pharmacological literature', *Canadian Journal of Physiology and Pharmacology*, **64**, 1.

Smith, D. A. and Cole, W. J., (1976), 'Identification of an arylesterase as the enzyme hydrolysing diacetylmorphine (heroin) in human plasma', *Biochemical Pharmacology*, **25**, 367.

Twycross, R. G., Fry, D. E. and Wills, P. D., (1974), 'The alimentary absorption of diamorphine and morphine in man as indicated by urinary excretion studies', *British Journal of Clinical Pharmacology*, **1**, 491.

Umans, J. G. and Inturrisi, G. E., (1982), 'Heroin: analgesia, toxicity and disposition in mouse', *European Journal of Pharmacology*, **85**, 317.

Umans, J. G., Chiu, T. S. K., Lipman, R. A., Schultz, M. F., Shin, S-U. and Inturrisi, C. E., (1982), 'Determination of heroin and its metabolites by high performance liquid chromatography', *Journal of Chromatography*, **233**, 213.

Van Steenberge, A., (1985), 'Epidural lofentanil for pain relief in labour', *Anaesthezie Intenzivmedicin*, **31**, 394.

Watson, J., Moore, A., McQuay, H., Teddy, P., Baldwin, D., Allen, M. and Bullingham, R., (1984), 'Plasma morphine concentrations and analgesic effects of lumbar extradural morphine and heroin', *Anesthesia and Analgesia*, **63**, 629.

Way, E. L. and Adler, T. K., (1962), 'The biological disposition of morphine and its surrogates – 2', *Bulletin of the World Health Organisation*, **26**, 51.

Way, E. L., Kemp, J. W., Young, J. M. and Grassetti, D. R., (1960), 'The pharmacologic effects of heroin in relationship to its rate of biotransformation', *Journal of Pharmacology and Experimental Therapeutics*, **129**, 144.

Way, E. L., Young, J. M. and Kemp, J. W., (1965), 'Metabolism of heroin and its pharmacological implications', *Bulletin of Narcotics*, **17**, 25.

Williams, F. M., (1985), 'Clinical significance of esterases in man', *Clinical Pharmacokinetics*, **10**, 392.

World Health Organisation, (1974), 'Detection of dependence-producing drugs in body fluids', in *Technical Report Series No. 556*, (Geneva, WHO).

Wright, C. I., (1942), 'The deacetylation of heroin and related compounds by mammalian tissues', *Journal of Pharmacology and Experimental Therapeutics*, **75**, 328.

Wright, B. M. and Callan, K., (1979), 'Slow drug infusions using a portable syringe drive', *British Medical Journal*, **ii**, 582.

Yeh, S. Y., Gorodetzky, C. W. and McQuinn, R. L., (1976), 'Urinary excretion of heroin and its metabolites in man', *Journal of Pharmacology and Experimental Therapeutics*, **126**, 249.

Yeh, S. Y., McQuinn, R. L. and Gorodetzky, C. W., (1977), 'Identification of diacetylmorphine metabolites in humans', *Journal of Pharmacological Sciences*, **66**, 201.

PROFESSOR CHRISTOPHER J. HULL, FFARCS

3 The pharmacodynamics of diamorphine

Following synthesis by C. R. A. Wright in 1874, diamorphine was first marketed commercially by the Bayer Company in 1898 as a powerful cough suppressant. Today, this might seem inappropriate since other drugs, such as codeine, are both effective and less prone to troublesome side-effects. However, it must be remembered that in the late nineteenth century tuberculosis was commonplace and cough suppressants more powerful than codeine found ready application, especially when the problem of dependence was, as yet, unrecognized. When it became apparent that dependence was a feature of prolonged morphine administration, diamorphine was, for a time, promoted as a safer substitute. Experience soon showed this not to be the case. The analgesic properties of diamorphine are long-established, and remain the sole reason for its continued use. As will be detailed below, it has some advantages over morphine in that it can be administered by a variety of routes and has shorter onset latency and greater subjective effects. These features have led a number of clinicians to regard diamorphine as being especially useful in the management of pain in the terminally ill. With the recent surge of interest in the intraspinal route (both subarachnoid and epidural) of administration, the unique physicochemical characteristics of diamorphine have led to new applications in the management of acute pain, especially that following surgery. North American patients are denied the benefit of this most effective drug since its manufacture is prohibited by Federal Law. However, prohibition appears to have done nothing to prevent its illicit use, and European experience has shown that diamorphine prepared for clinical use is no more likely to be misappropriated than other drugs of addiction.

The properties of diamorphine after intramuscular injection

In many respects diamorphine is very similar to morphine. However, it is more potent and has a different time-course of action.

Potency and time-profile

Foldes and his colleagues (Foldes, Swerdlow and Siker, 1964) estimated diamorphine to be 2–3.3 times more potent than morphine in man. In approximately equipotent doses, the effects of diamorphine both appear and wane more rapidly than those of morphine.

Subjective effects

Diamorphine causes mental clouding, euphoria and talkativeness, but with reduced friendliness to others. The impairment of mental performance has been reported to be one of speed rather than accuracy (Smith, Semke and Beecher, 1962). Following equianalgesic doses, the subjective effects of diamorphine have been reported to develop more quickly and have greater intensity than those of morphine (Smith and Beecher, 1962). However, Dundee's group found no significant differences in the frequency or intensity of subjective effects when given before anaesthesia, but did report that the effects following diamorphine were of shorter duration than those of morphine (Dundee, Loan and Clarke, 1966).

Analgesia

Diamorphine is a powerful narcotic analgesic, with 5 mg roughly equivalent to morphine 10 mg (Dundee, Loan and Clarke, 1966; Jacobson *et al.*, 1983). However, other workers have found diamorphine 5 mg to be an unsatisfactory analgesic in the early postoperative period after major abdominal surgery, with a duration of action rarely exceeding 90 minutes (Malins *et al.*, 1984).

The analgesic effect has two components; a rather weak effect in reducing the intensity of painful sensations and a much more powerful effect in increasing the capacity to tolerate those sensations. Indeed, a suitable dose is capable of transforming a frightened, suffering creature into a calm, stoic patient with a marked sense of well-being.

Respiratory depression and cough suppression

Diamorphine causes respiratory depression in a similar manner to morphine. The primary effect is to reduce the responsiveness of the respiratory centres to CO_2, but large doses will also depress responsiveness to hypoxia and lead to life-threatening hypoventilation.

Malins and his colleagues studied the effects of intramuscular diamorphine 5 mg on minute volume and the ventilatory response to CO_2 (Malins *et al.*, 1984). After 30 minutes minute volume was reduced by 17 per cent and CO_2 response by 33 per cent. At 90 minutes the reductions were 20 per cent and 37 per cent, and by 90 minutes had started to recover. Clearly, there is considerable overlap between the analgesic and respiratory depressant effects of diamorphine, and it is certain that an effective analgesic dose will cause measurable respiratory depression.

Diamorphine suppresses cough by a direct effect upon the cough centre in the medulla. This action is quite independent of the respiratory depressant effects. It is often claimed that diamorphine is a more powerful cough suppressant than morphine, but in common with many other aspects of this drug's pharmacological profile, hard evidence is in short supply.

Cardiovascular effects

As with morphine, diamorphine in high dosage causes bradycardia as a result of increased vagal activity and reduced sympathetic activity. Similarly, it causes widespread vasodilatation which may lead to modest reductions in arterial blood pressure. However, normal analgesic doses (2–5 mg in adults) have little or no cardiovascular effects. In those subjects in whom a euphoriant effect is produced, catecholamine release may cause a transient increase in both blood pressure and heart rate.

Seizure activity

Like all other strong opioids, diamorphine can cause convulsions and EEG seizure activity when given in high dosage (Volavka *et al.*, 1970).

Gastrointestinal effects

Diamorphine causes the same range of gastro-intestinal effects as morphine. Gastric motility and acid secretion are reduced, and gastric emptying is prolonged. Biliary and pancreatic secretions are markedly diminished, the tone of the sphincter of Oddi is increased and biliary tract pressure is increased. Small intestinal tone is increased, but there is a reduction in propulsive activity. Similarly, propulsive activity in the colon is reduced, but resting tone is greatly increased, almost to the point of spasm.

Anal sphincteric tone is increased. This effect, together with faecal desiccation due to prolonged transit-time and the loss of voiding urgency associated with the central action of diamorphine, causes severe constipation. However, there is an unconfirmed clinical impression that it causes *less* constipation than morphine in equianalgesic doses (Twycross, 1973).

Effects on other smooth muscle

In large doses, diamorphine may cause bronchoconstriction. Both tone and contractions of the ureters are increased. Similarly, the tone of the detrusor and vesical sphincter muscles are increased, leading in some patients to urinary retention. In therapeutic doses, diamorphine has little effect on the uterus.

Nausea and vomiting

In some, but not all subjects, diamorphine stimulates the Chemoreceptor Trigger Zone (CTZ) in the *area postrema* of the medulla to cause nausea and vomiting. However, there is a widely held impression that diamorphine causes less nausea or vomiting than does morphine in equianalgesic doses. However, firm evidence is, as yet, lacking.

Most opioids are, despite their stimulant effects upon the CTZ, anti-emetics as a result of direct depressant effects upon the vomiting centre itself; this can be demonstrated as inhibition of apomorphine-induced vomiting. This effect has not been demonstrated for diamorphine, but should be assumed to occur until shown otherwise.

Miosis

Diamorphine causes miosis with a similar time course to that of morphine, with approximately twice the potency (Nutt and Jasinski, 1973).

Effects on the skin

Like morphine, diamorphine causes widespread vasodilatation, mild diaphoresis and piloerection. This may be accompanied by itching, which can be severe in a small proportion of cases. The causation of itching is uncertain, but may be associated with histamine release.

Tolerance, dependence and abuse potential

As with all other strong agonist opioids, the dosage of regularly administered diamorphine may be escalated rapidly to very high levels. For instance, Martin and Fraser showed that the daily dose could be increased from 13 mg to 87 mg in only 20 days (Martin and Fraser, 1961). Similarly, they showed that morphine dosage could be increased from 30 to 207 mg daily over the same period. On withdrawal, both groups of subjects developed abstinence syndromes of similar intensity, with those in the morphine group persisting somewhat longer. They concluded that equipotent doses of morphine and diamorphine had identical potential for both tolerance and physical dependence. Continued administration to patients with terminal pain may necessitate steady increases in dosage; so much so that daily consumption may reach 2 g or more.

The possibility that diamorphine may lead to acute tolerance (i.e., within a few hours) has not been investigated in any depth. However, a study of diamorphine given by continuous intravenous infusion to 'volunteers' showed no evidence of acute tolerance developing within 7 hours (Elliott *et al.*, 1971).

Spinal and epidural administration

In 1976 Yaksh and Rudy showed that opioids injected directly into the CSF caused profound analgesia in rats. Since that discovery, there has been increasing enthusiasm for both spinal and epidural administration of opioids in the management of severe pain. It was inevitable that diamorphine would not escape attention. In fact, these techniques have given a new lease of life to a drug whose fortunes were, until recently, subsiding slowly into obscurity.

Given in the same dose range as intramuscular injection (adult dose 5 mg), epidural diamorphine produces useful analgesia within 10–15 minutes (Jacobson *et al.*, 1983). This rapid onset contrasts sharply with the 30–60 minute onset times observed with morphine (Bromage, Camporesi and Chestnut, 1980). The duration of action is very variable, ranging from 2 to 21 hours. By comparison with intramuscular injection, urinary retention and pruritus occur more commonly. Diamorphine is absorbed into the bloodstream from the epidural space much more rapidly than morphine; so much so that systemic side-effects such as respiratory depression are likely to follow large doses. Indeed, a comparative study of epidural and IM diamorphine concluded that the former route is simply an exotic means of delivering diamorphine to the brain (Jacobson *et al.*, 1983). However, whereas morphine has been reported to cause *late* respiratory depression (Reiz *et al.*, 1981; Weddel and Ritter, 1981) 6–10 hours after epidural administration, presumably due to rostral spread within the CSF, this complication has not been reported following epidural diamorphine.

Much smaller doses (1–2 mg) are effective when administered directly into the CSF, and have a more predictable duration of action, ranging from 12 to 25 hours (Paterson *et al.*, 1984). As with epidural administration, nausea, pruritus and retention are common side-effects. Whereas intrathecal morphine in small (1 mg) doses has been shown to cause late, severe respiratory depression (Davies, Tolhurst-Cleaver and James, 1980), this complication has not been reported with diamorphine. Diamorphine is taken up into the bloodstream much more rapidly than morphine, but by virtue of the very small (1–2 mg) doses given, is most unlikely to cause complications of any kind.

Other routes of administration

Diamorphine is well absorbed from the gastrointestinal tract, but is subject to extensive first-pass metabolism and therefore appears to be less potent when taken by this route. Since it is readily absorbed from oral or nasal mucosae, the venous drainage of which does not lead to the liver, diamorphine may be administered quite efficiently in the form of snuff or sublingual tablets.

The mode of action of diamorphine

The pharmacological properties of diamorphine are directly related to its physicochemical properties and disposition within the body. Since many of these features are considered in some detail in separate chapters, this account serves only to explain the unique mode of action of diamorphine in terms of fundamental principles.

Physicochemical properties

Diamorphine is the 3, 6, diacetyl derivative of morphine. Like morphine it is a weak base, with a pKa value of 7.83. Thus at pH 7.4, 73 per cent is protonated and 27 per cent unionised base. As might be expected, the protonated form is hydrophilic and very poorly lipid soluble, but the free base is much more lipid soluble than that of morphine. At pH 7.4 the heptane:water partition coefficients for diamorphine and morphine are 0.043 and 0.00006 respectively. Although more lipid soluble than morphine, diamorphine should not really be classed as a lipid-soluble opioid; it is, for instance, 440 times *less* lipid soluble than fentanyl, whose heptane:water partition coefficient at pH 7.4 is 19. However, since 60 per cent of plasma diamorphine is unbound (fentanyl 16 per cent) and of that fraction some 27 per cent is free base (fentanyl 9 per cent), the 'diffusible fraction' amounts to some 16 per cent (fentanyl 1.4 per cent). This greater diffusible fraction has no influence upon blood:tissue partition *at equilibrium*, but does imply that diamorphine will diffuse across lipid cell membranes 11 times more rapidly than would be expected from a simple consideration of lipid solubility alone.

Deacetylation of diamorphine

Diamorphine is deacetylated rapidly by esterases (in blood and a variety of tissues) to 6-O-acetylmorphine (6-AM) and then morphine (Way *et al.*, 1960; Way *et al.*, 1965; Lockridge *et al.*, 1980). It is of some interest to note that in *plasma*, diamorphine is deacetylated by serum cholinesterase

(Inturrisi *et al.*, 1983) and therefore may become involved in pharmacokinetic interactions with other drugs (such as suxamethonium) which depend upon that enzyme for their degradation. At least three distinct enzymes within the red blood cell are capable of deacetylating diamorphine (Owen and Nakatsu, 1982), while in the central nervous system other, as yet unidentified esterases are involved. Gianutsos and his colleagues (1986) have shown that both peripheral and central esterases are important in converting diamorphine into its active metabolites. Although diamorphine hydrolyses spontaneously in alkaline solutions (Oberst, 1943), this does not occur to any measurable extent at physiological pH (Nakamura, Thornton and Naguchi, 1975).

Hydrolysis of 6-AM to morphine occurs predominantly in the liver, where glucuronidation represents the main excretion pathway (Boerner, Abbott and Roe, 1975).

Receptor binding of diamorphine and its metabolites

Since it is accepted that an unsubstituted phenolic hydroxyl group at the 3-position is essential for opioid receptor binding, 3-6-diacetyl morphine would not be expected to be active, and indeed it is not. In fact, diamorphine is a prodrug, and as such does not bind to opioid receptors and has no intrinsic opioid activity (Inturrisi *et al.*, 1983). The first metabolite 6-AM *does* bind to opioid μ receptors (Inturrisi *et al.*, 1983), and has been widely assumed to be responsible for at least the initial phase of the observed pharmacological effect (Eddy and Howes, 1935; Way *et al.*, 1965). Since high concentrations can be demonstrated in CSF, and receptor binding undoubtedly occurs, this may indeed be the case. However, although 6-AM can displace naloxone from opioid receptor sites, this does *not* show that it thereby exerts a pharmacological effect; there is no direct evidence to show that 6-AM possesses intrinsic opioid activity.

Von Cube and his colleagues showed that morphine is 900 times more potent when injected directly into brain-CSF than when administered intravenously (Von Cube *et al.*, 1970). This suggests that the diamorphine which diffuses rapidly into the brain substance and there dissociates into 6-AM might well, in fact, yield sufficient morphine to exert the initial effect. This possibility is supported by the 'rush' effect, by which an intensely pleasurable sensation very rapidly follows intravenous injection; this could *only* occur if diamorphine penetrates the brain substance before deacetylation to non-lipid-soluble products (Martin and Fraser, 1961). Since it is currently impossible to study the pharmacological effects of 6-AM without concurrent deacetylation to morphine, this point must remain unresolved. However, it *is* safe to assume that the late effects of diamorphine are due to the actions of morphine upon (predominantly) μ receptors, since 6-AM concentrations decay to very low levels *before* the termination of effect.

Mode of action of diamorphine after intramuscular injection

As may be expected from a much more lipid-soluble substance, diamorphine is absorbed from injection sites much more rapidly than morphine. Upon reaching the bloodstream, heroin is converted to 6-AM with a half-time of 9 minutes (Nakamura, Thornton and Naguchi, 1975). In turn, 6-AM hydrolyses to morphine, but with a half-time approaching 1 hour. Both products are very much less lipid soluble. As might be expected, diamorphine distributes rapidly to other tissues. Consequently the plasma concentration of unchanged diamorphine decays very rapidly indeed with a half time of less than 5 minutes (Umans *et al.*, 1982). Thus we may see diamorphine not so much as a drug but as a delivery system; it crosses lipid membranes such as the blood-brain barrier freely and therefore reaches opioid receptor sites in neural tissues much more rapidly and completely than does morphine (Oldendorf *et al.*, 1972). The studies carried out by Oldendorf's group are of particular interest; they measured the extraction of morphine and diamorphine from the carotid arteries of rats and found that whereas 1.5 per cent of morphine was extracted in a single pass, 65 per cent of diamorphine was removed (Oldendorf *et al.*, 1972).

It is not surprising to find pharmacological differences between morphine and diamorphine as well as differences in the rates of onset; these may simply reflect different patterns of penetration to target sites within the brain. At these sites of action, transformation to morphine (which crosses lipid membranes slowly) leads to more sustained effects than would be expected from a lipid-soluble agent. Of course, the diamorphine which is deacetylated in plasma behaves as morphine in every major respect.

Mode of action of intrathecal diamorphine

When diamorphine is placed in the CSF it exerts its pharmacological effect by diffusion into the substance of the spinal cord. Rapid deacetylation to 6-AM and then morphine is followed by receptor occupancy; mostly to μ receptors in the *substantia gelatinosa*. In contrast to plasma, CSF contains no enzymes capable of deacetylating diamorphine.

At the same time, diamorphine is absorbed into the bloodstream from both CSF and neural tissues themselves, thereby leading to systemic effects. However, since the administered dose is very small (1–2 mg) these effects are likely to be minimal (see Fig. 2.5).

Since systemic uptake of unchanged diamorphine is very rapid, only part of the administered dose reaches the cord substance in any form. However, that small fraction delivers morphine directly to the sites of action and thereby causes the spinal effects, presumably by occupancy of μ receptors which are present in abundance in the *substantia gelatinosa*. Once within the substance of the cord, morphine diffuses out very slowly by virtue of its very low lipid solubility. Thus analgesia of extended duration may be achieved.

By contrast with intrathecal morphine (Gustafsson, Schildt and Jacobsen, 1982), *late* respiratory depression has not been reported after intrathecal diamorphine. This is to be expected, since uptake of diamorphine by neural structures is much greater than that of morphine, and the morphine which evolves *from* that diamorphine is released into the CSF very slowly indeed. In consequence, the amount of morphine available for rostral spread is very limited and most unlikely to cause serious side-effects. This contrasts with the behaviour of intrathecal morphine, where much of the administered dose remains free within the CSF and subject to unpredictable bulk movement which may reach the basal cisterna within 3 hours (Max *et al.*, 1985).

Mode of action of epidural diamorphine

When diamorphine is placed in the epidural space, it exerts its pharmacological effect by diffusion into the CSF and then the substance of the spinal cord.

At the same time, diamorphine is absorbed into the bloodstream from both epidural space and CSF, thereby leading to the full range of systemic effects. It is likely that only a small fraction of the administered diamorphine reaches the cord substance in any form. However, that small fraction delivers morphine directly to the site of action and thereby causes the spinal effects. Since diamorphine diffuses easily across the 'blood-brain barrier', the only impediment in this process is the dura itself. Moore and his colleagues have shown that whereas morphine and diamorphine have very similar permeabilities, fentanyl is 4 times more permeable (Moore *et al.*, 1982). However, it has been suggested that the main route of CSF uptake from the epidural space may well be through the dural cuff region (Modig and Paalzow, 1981).

By contrast with epidural morphine, *late* respiratory depression has not been reported after epidural diamorphine. As with the spinal route, this is to be expected. First, the mass of morphine yielded by an effective dose of diamorphine is less than half that which must be given as morphine itself. Second, as before, uptake of diamorphine by neural tissues is much greater than that of morphine, and is released into the CSF very slowly.

References

Boerner, U., Abbott, S. and Roe, R. L., (1978), 'The metabolism of morphine and heroin in man', *Drug Metabolism Reviews*, **4**, 39.

Bromage, P. R., Camporesi, E. and Chestnut, D., (1980), 'Epidural narcotics for postoperative analgesia', *Anesthesia and Analgesia*, **59**, 473.

Davies, G. K., Tolhurst-Cleaver, C. L. and James, T. L., (1980), 'Respiratory depression after intrathecal narcotics', *Anaesthesia*, **35**, 1,080.

Dundee, J. W., Loan, W. B., and Clarke, R. S. J., (1966), 'Studies of drugs given before anaesthesia. XI. diamorphine (heroin) and morphine', *British Journal of Anaesthesia*, **38**, 610.

Eddy, N. B. and Howes, H. A., (1935), 'Studies of morphine, codeine and their derivatives. VIII. Monoacetyl- and diacetylmorphine and their hydrogenated derivatives', *Journal of Pharmacology and Experimental Therapeutics*, **53**, 430.

Elliott, H. W., Parker, K. D., Wright, J. A. and Nomof, N., (1971), 'Actions and metabolism of heroin administered by continuous infusion to man', *Clinical Pharmacology and Therapeutics*, **12**, 806.

Foldes, F. F., Swerdlow, M. and Siker, E. S., (1964), in *Narcotics and narcotic antagonists*, (Springfield, Illinois: Thomas, Charles C., 1st edition).

Gianutsos, G., Cohen, S. D., Carlson, G., Heyman, R., Salva, P., Morrow, G. and Hite, G. J., (1986), 'Alteration of in vivo and in vitro effects of heroin by esterase inhibition', *Toxicology and Applied Pharmacology*, **82**, 14.

Gustafsson, L. L., Schildt, B. and Jacobsen, K. J., (1982), 'Adverse effects of extradural and intrathecal opiates: report of a nationwide survey in Sweden', *British Journal of Anaesthesia*, **54**, 479.

Inturrisi, C. E., Schultz, M., Shin, S., Umans, J. G., Angel, L. and Simon, E. J., (1983), 'Evidence from binding studies that heroin acts through its metabolites', *Life Sciences*, **33** (suppl. II), 773.

Jacobson, L., Phillips, P. D., Hull, C. J. and Conacher, I. D., (1983), 'Extradural versus intramuscular diamorphine. A controlled study of analgesic and adverse effects in the postoperative period', *Anaesthesia*, **38**, 10.

Kotob, H. I. M., Hand, C. W., Moore, R. A., Evans, P. J. D., Wells, J., Rubin, A. P. and McQuay, H. J., (1986), 'Intrathecal morphine and heroin in humans. 6-hour drug levels in spinal fluid and plasma', *Anesthesia and Analgesia*, **65**, 718.

Lockridge, O., Mottershaw-Jackson, N., Eckerson, H. W. and La Du B. N., (1980), 'Hydrolysis of diacetyl morphine (heroin) by human serum cholinesterase', *Journal of Pharmacology and Experimental Therapeutics*, **215**, 1.

Malins, A. F., Goodman, N. W., Cooper, G. M., Prys-Roberts, C. and Baird, R. N., (1984), 'Ventilatory effects of pre- and postoperative diamorphine', *Anaesthesia*, **39**, 118.

Martin, W. R. and Fraser, H. F., (1961), 'A comparative study of physiological and subjective effects of heroin and morphine administered intravenously in post-addicts', *Journal of Pharmacology and Experimental Therapeutics*, **133**, 388.

Max, M. B., Inturrisi, C. E., Kaiko, R. F., Grabinski, P. Y., Li, C.H. and Foley, K. M., (1985), 'Epidural and intrathecal opiates: cerebrospinal fluid and plasma profiles in cancer pain patients', *Clinical Pharmacology and Therapeutics* **38**, 631.

Modig, J. and Paalzow, L., (1981), 'A comparison of epidural morphine and epidural bupivacaine for postoperative pain relief', *Acta Anaesthesiologica Scandinavica*, **25**, 437.

Moore, R. A., Bullingham, R. E. S., McQuay, H. J., Hand, C. W., Aspel, J. B., Allen, M. C. and Thomas, D., (1982), 'Dural permeability to narcotics: in vitro determination and application to extradural administration', *British Journal of Anaesthesia*, **54**, 1,117.

Nakamura, G. R., Thornton, J. and Noguchi, T. T., (1975), 'Kinetics of heroin deacetylation in aqueous alkaline solution and in human serum and whole blood', *Journal of Chromatography*, **110**, 81.

Nutt, J. C. and Jasinski, D. R., (1973), 'Comparison of intravenously administered methadone, morphine, heroin and placebo', *Federation Proceedings*, **32**, 694.

Oberst, F. W., (1943), 'Studies on the fate of heroin', *Journal of Pharmacology and Experimental Therapeutics*, **79**, 266.

Oldendorf, W. H., Hyman, S., Braun, L. and Oldendorf, S. Z., (1972), 'Blood-brain barrier penetration of morphine, codeine, heroin and methadone after carotid injection', *Science*, **178**, 984.

Owen, J. A. and Nakatsu, K., (1982), 'Diacetylmorphine (heroin) hydrolases in human blood', *Canadian Journal of Physiology and Pharmacology*, **61**, 870.

Paterson, G. M. C., McQuay, H. J., Bullingham, R. E. S. and Moore, R. A., (1984), 'Intradural morphine and diamorphine. Dose response studies', *Anaesthesia*, **39**, 113.

Reiz, S., Ahlin, J., Ahrenfeld, B. and Andersson, M., (1981), 'Epidural morphine for postoperative pain relief', *Acta Anaesthesiologica Scandinavica*, **25**, 111.

Smith, G. M. and Beecher, H. K., (1962), 'Subjective effects of heroin and morphine in normal subjects', *Journal of Pharmacology and Experimental Therapeutics*, **136**, 47.

Smith, G. M., Semke, C. W. and Beecher, H. K., (1962), 'Objective evidence of mental effects of heroin and morphine and placebo in normal subjects', *Journal of Pharmacology and Experimental Therapeutics*, **136**, 53.

Twycross, R. G., (1973), 'Stumbling blocks in the study of diamorphine', *Postgraduate Medical Journal*, **49**, 309.

Umans, J. G., Chiu, T. S. K., Lipman, R. A., Schultz, M. F., Shin, S. and Inturissi, C. E., (1982), 'Determination of heroin and its metabolites by high performance liquid chromatography', *Journal of Chromatography*, **233**, 213.

Volavka, J., Zaks, A., Roubicek, J. and Fink, M., (1970), 'Electrographic effects of diacetyl morphine (heroin) and naloxone in man', *Neuropharmacology*, **9**, 587.

Von Cube, B., Teschemacher, H. J., Hertz, A. and Hess, R., (1970), 'Permeation of morphine-like acting substances to their sites of anti-nociceptive action in the brain after intravenous and intraventricular application and dependence upon lipid-solubility', *Naunyn-Schmiedebergs Archives of Pharmacology*, **265**, 455.

Way, E. L., Kemp, J. W., Young, J. M. and Grassetti, D. R., (1960), 'The pharmacologic effects of heroin in relationship to its rate of biotransformation', *Journal of Pharmacology and Experimental Therapeutics*, **129**, 144.

Way, E. L., Young, J. M. and Kemp, J. W., (1965), 'Metabolism of heroin and its pharmacological implications', *Bulletin of Narcotics*, **17**, 25.

Weddel, S. J. and Ritter, R. R., (1981), 'Serum levels following epidural administration of morphine and correlation with relief of post surgical pain', *Anesthesiology*, **54**, 210.

Yaksh, T. L. and Rudy, T. A., (1976), 'Analgesia mediated by a direct spinal effect of narcotics', *Science*, **192**, 1,357.

D. BRUCE SCOTT, MD, FRCPE, FFARCS

4 The use of diamorphine in acute pain

Opioids, morphine in particular, have held a central and pre-eminent place in the alleviation of acute pain for centuries. Their effectiveness is undoubted and, paradoxically, they have suffered from their own success in that their prescription tends to be automatic and routine, resulting in analgesia that is often much less than optimal and, conversely, is occasionally associated with serious side-effects.

While the relief of acute pain is a major clinical objective, the use of opioids has certain constraints which must be understood. These include the following:

1. The avoidance of overdosage and particularly the development of respiratory inadequacy.
2. The need for the cause of the pain to be accurately diagnosed. In conditions such as an acute abdomen, total relief of the pain may interfere with the clinical picture. Having said that, the clinician should not use this as an excuse for delaying analgesia unnecessarily. It is difficult to overestimate the pain caused by conditions such as acute colic due to gallstones or renal stones.
3. The recognition that the sedation, which accompanies analgesia to a greater or lesser extent, may occasionally be undesirable, for example, in the assessment of the progress of a head injury.

Advantages of diamorphine

Diamorphine is an excellent drug in acute pain management. Due to its pharmacokinetic behaviour it achieves a more rapid effect than morphine

(Kaiko *et al.*, 1981). Its much greater lipid solubility and that of its metabolite, monoacetylmorphine, allows it to reach its target receptors in the brain more quickly than is the case with morphine. It is more rapidly absorbed from subcutaneous and intramuscular injection sites.

In the United Kingdom it is one of the most commonly used opioids for acute pain relief. Unfortunately there are few, if any, convincing comparative trials of the various opioids in this field (Levine *et al.*, 1986). However, the reasons for using the drug in preference to morphine are many, some based on good scientific evidence but most on clinical experience, a notoriously fickle method of judgement. Nevertheless, the following are the reasons given by clinicians for preferring diamorphine:

1. It is twice as potent as morphine.
2. Its action is faster.
3. It causes less nausea and vomiting.
4. It has a more pleasant psychic effect than morphine, a drug often associated with depression. The validity of this would be indicated by the fact that addicts much prefer it to morphine. The possibility of addicting a patient by using the drug to relieve pain is mentioned below.
5. Its cardiovascular effects are less than those of morphine and it has been recommended for the relief of pain in acute myocardial infarction (Macdonald *et al.*, 1967; Scott and Orr, 1969).

Disadvantages of diamorphine

1. It is said to be more addictive than morphine. Certainly heroin addiction is nowadays much more common than morphine addiction, but there is little or no difference in the rate at which dependence develops to either drug. The popularity of heroin among addicts almost certainly relates to the difference in degree and speed of onset of its psychic effects, particularly euphoria, and to its solubility which allows large doses to be dissolved in small volumes of water.

   Though a theoretical risk, the development of addiction to opioids used to relieve acute pain is extremely uncommon. Even when used for chronic or terminal pain, craving for the drug is not evident, though tolerance is usually evident after 1 to 2 weeks. This presumably relates to the motivation in taking the drug which is completely different in an addict who wishes to achieve a 'high' and a patient with severe pain who wants relief from that pain.

2. Its duration of effect is shorter (by about 25%) than morphine.
3. Its bad reputation in regard to addiction often leads to a negative attitude on the part of doctors who prescribe, and nurses who administer, diamorphine.

Ineffective use of opioids

Morphine or diamorphine can, in a non-tolerant individual, virtually always totally relieve acute pain if given in sufficient dosage by an appropriate route. In spite of this, inadequate pain relief is probably as common, if not commoner, than adequate pain relief. The reasons for this are many but they include the following:

1. Patient variability. Pain is completely subjective and only the patient can judge the adequacy of analgesia. The dose of drug-producing analgesia can vary very much from patient to patient (Mather and Phillips, 1986). Moreover pain varies in degree and duration according to the condition causing it. Thus the pain of labour can be one of the most severe kinds of pain and is not comparable to traumatic pain. The prescription of a standard dose, given at a standard site, and to be repeated after a standard interval (e.g., morphine 10 mg IM 4-hourly) will be inadequate in many patients, and may be too much for others.

2. The result of the initial injection is seldom seriously enquired into at the time, and the necessary dosage adjustment is often not made.

3. Too little drug is prescribed. This, no doubt, is due to fear by doctors of respiratory depression which can be fatal, while pain, of itself is not lethal.

4. The drug is not given as prescribed. Nurses are notoriously unwilling to give repeat doses. This is probably related to the unwarranted fear that addiction will develop. The use of 'p.r.n.' on a prescription will almost always be interpreted as 'never more frequently than 4-hourly (or longer)'. Diamorphine given intramuscularly seldom lasts longer than 3 hours and prolonged painful intervals can occur between injections.

5. The duration of pain is variable and if prolonged beyond the normal course, as may easily happen in, say, postoperative pain, recourse to less effective drugs is made.

Optimal use of opioids in acute pain

The clinician must decide on the drug, the dose, the route and the frequency of administration in relation to the circumstances in which the drug is being given. Clearly the use of an opioid at the site of a road accident will be quite different from its administration in hospital. It must be obvious that to obtain optimal results, the drug and dosage must be fitted to the patient and not vice versa.

Routes of injection

The use of oral opioids, so valuable in treating chronic pain, is of little value in acute pain. Therefore the drugs must be injected.

Subcutaneous injection has no place in the treatment of acute pain as the absorption from this site is extremely variable, skin-blood flow being dependent upon body temperature and the degree of sympathetic activity in the presence of pain, apprehension and clinically obvious shock.

Intramuscular injection is the commonest route of injection but it also has considerable variations in absorption rate, even in the same patient, albeit less than with subcutaneous injection. After pethidine 100 mg IM, peak plasma concentrations were reached at times varying from 20–100 min and at levels of 0.25 to 0.63 mg/l (Mather *et al.*, 1975). The big advantage of this route is its simplicity and convenience, especially if given by the nursing staff.

Intravenous injection is the most effective method of giving opioid because the plasma concentration can be increased rapidly and maintained at an effective level. However, it requires a doctor who is prepared to stay with the patient until the effect has been properly assessed and the maintenance dose calculated. It can be used to obtain initial analgesia, any subsequent dose being given intramuscularly.

   Fortunately with diamorphine, the effect is rapid and therefore easier to assess than with some other opioids. Nevertheless the initial dose must be given slowly to avoid overdosage. Maintenance of the analgesia can be by repeated intravenous injections, a continuous infusion, or by a patient-operated pump. Choosing the appropriate method for an individual patient requires consideration of the plasma concentrations of opioid produced by these regimes.

Intraspinal injection. This is dealt with in Chapter 6 (see page 82).

Plasma concentrations

For each patient there will be a minimum effective analgesic plasma concentration (which will depend upon the pain intensity) and a toxic plasma concentration at which respiratory depression will occur. The aim of therapy is to achieve a plasma concentration between these two (Fig. 4.1), and to maintain it there for as long as necessary. As mentioned in previous chapters, diamorphine is metabolised to monoacetyl morphine, and then to morphine, both of which are active analgesics. As morphine concentrations are easily measured, compared to diamorphine or mono-acetylmorphine, only morphine concentrations will be described here for the sake of clarity.

Intermittent injections will cause the plasma concentration to rise and fall, risking both over- and under-dosage (Figs 4.2 and 4.3). These can only be avoided by the frequent injection of doses which are insufficient to reach the toxic level, bearing in mind that at the time of each injection the concentration will not usually have returned to zero (Fig. 4.4).

Intravenously, a loading dose will raise the plasma concentration rapidly into the effective range (Fig. 4.5). It can be maintained in this range

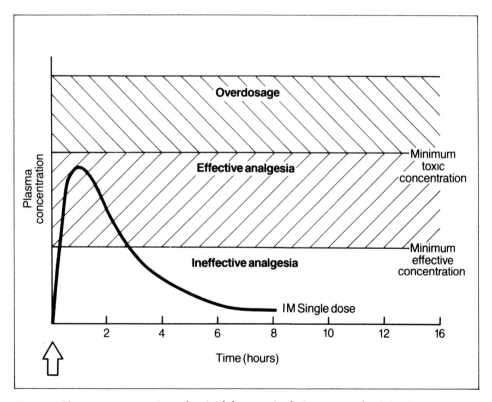

Fig. 4.1 Plasma concentration of opioid from a single intramuscular injection.

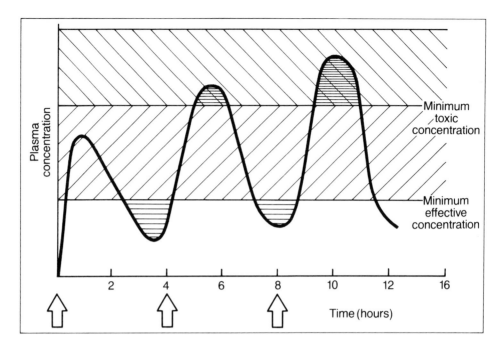

Fig. 4.2 Plasma concentration of opioid following repeated intramuscular dosage at 4-hourly intervals. There is a tendency for periods of overdosage and ineffective analgesia to occur.

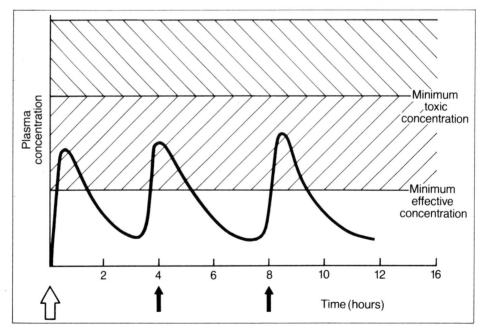

Fig. 4.3 Plasma concentration of opioid with small intramuscular doses given 4-hourly.

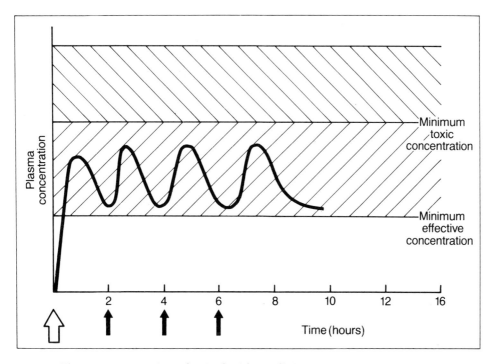

Fig. 4.4 Plasma concentration of opioid with small doses given 2-hourly.

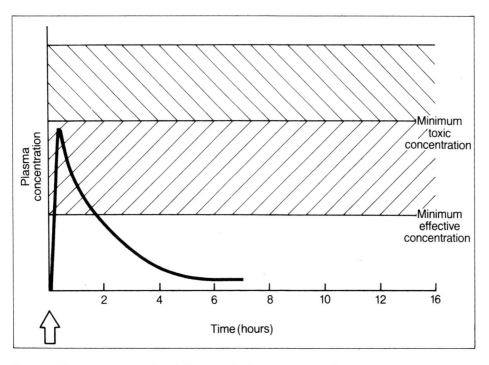

Fig. 4.5 Plasma concentration following single intravenous dose.

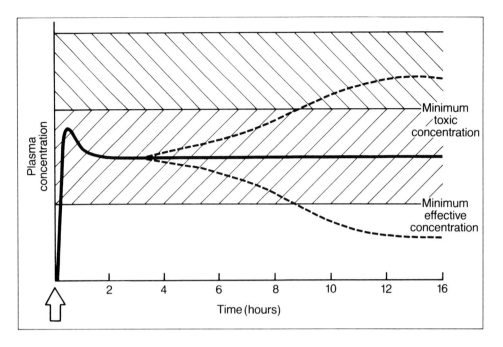

Fig. 4.6 Plasma concentration following initial intravenous loading dose, plus a continuous infusion. Dotted lines represent concentrations if the infusion is too fast (upper line) or too slow (lower line).

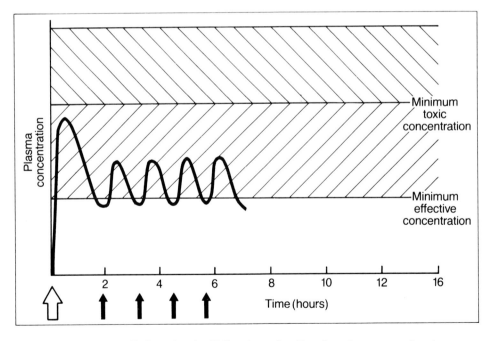

Fig. 4.7 Patient-controlled analgesia. Following a loading dose intravenously, the patient triggers a small intravenous injection whenever analgesia is required.

by an infusion (Fig. 4.6). However the infusion may cause the concentration to rise steadily (if more is injected than is metabolised) and exceed the toxic level. Conversely the concentration may fall below the effective level.

It is possible to use specially-designed pumps that will inject intravenously, in small doses predetermined by the clinician, when the pump is activated by the patient. Thus, every time the patient feels pain, he/she may inject a further dose and re-establish an effective plasma concentration (Fig. 4.7). The maximum frequency of repeat injections are also set by the clinician and this cannot be overridden by the patient (Evans *et al.*, 1978). This is referred to as 'patient-controlled analgesia', and it has the advantage of preventing overdosage while making full allowance for patient variation.

Dosage

Intramuscular

Diamorphine is usually given in a dose of 5 mg, though this should be decreased in the elderly, and may be increased in young patients with severe pain. Assessment of the effect after 30 to 60 minutes will allow a reasonable estimate of further dosage. If the patient has had no relief, a further 5 mg should be given. If some relief is achieved but is still not adequate, then 2.5 mg may be injected. If the patient is fully relieved but excessively drowsy, with a respiratory rate less than 12/min, then he/she should be carefully monitored and subsequent injections reduced to 2.5 mg.

Many dosage regimes calculate dosage on a body-weight basis. These should be treated with some suspicion, however, as they make the assumption that an overweight female is the same as a thin muscular male. Given the very large individual variations, it is advisable to keep the dosage simple, increasing or decreasing according to the clinical effect, and using body weight to calculate the dose only in children (0.1 mg/kg).

The frequency of injection is of great importance if painful hiatuses in analgesia are to be avoided. There is no logic whatever in the assumption that the effects of morphine, diamorphine and pethidine, all last 4 hours in all patients. Again only the patient can judge the effect and it is up to the doctor and/or nurse to decide on when a further injection is required. This may be after as little as 2 hours. It is, of course, quite possible to accumulate drug with frequent administration (Fig. 4.2), but it should be remembered that if reasonable analgesia was obtained with the previous injection, the reappearance of pain means the plasma concentration has decreased and further drug is required. P.r.n. does not mean 'not more frequently than 4-

hourly', it means exactly what it says, 'whenever necessary'. If accumulation is occurring, then the analgesia after each dose will last longer and the intervals between injections can be increased.

Intravenous

The intravenous administration of opioids has many advantages. Because analgesia will be rapid in onset, it allows the clinician to titrate the patient's need much more accurately. Moreover the administration can be maintained as a constant infusion leading to stable plasma concentrations, that is, a steady state is achieved. Alternatively, the injection of small boluses of opioid can be actuated by the patient, in the method called 'patient-controlled analgesia' (Harmer, Rosen and Vickers, 1985).

If the intravenous route is chosen, it will require more monitoring than is necessary with intramuscular opioid, particularly in regard to respiratory depression.

If diamorphine is used, 1 mg should be injected intravenously every 30 seconds until the patient's pain has clearly been relieved. This will usually take about 5–8 mg. If a continuous infusion is to follow this, then it should be at the rate of 25% of the initial effective bolus dose every hour, for example, if 6 mg were required to relieve the pain, then the continuous infusion should be at a rate of 1.5 mg/hr. Again the patient must be examined and questioned at frequent intervals and the dosage reviewed as necessary. With patient-controlled administration, the pump should be set to give 10% of the loading dose not more frequently than every 15 minutes, for example, if 6 mg was required to relieve pain, then the pump should be programmed to deliver doses of 0.6 mg at not less than 15-minute intervals.

Side-effects of diamorphine

While respiratory depression is the most dangerous side-effect, there are numerous others. Nausea and vomiting are very common with all opioids. Gastric emptying is greatly delayed (Nimmo *et al.*, 1975), and gut motility is depressed with resulting constipation. As diamorphine is metabolised to morphine it is almost certain that it has the same effect.

Pruritis and urinary retention can occur with most opioids but are seldom a problem unless the drugs are given epidurally or intrathecally.

Respiratory depression

This is the most important complication of diamorphine which, if the dosage is pushed, can cause respiratory arrest. The chief effect of opioids is to reduce the rate of respiration which is compensated for by an increase in the tidal volume. However, at respiratory rates of less than 10/min, some degree of hypercarbia and hypoxia are likely to occur. If the rate falls below 5/min it is usually accompanied by deep sedation with pin-point pupils, and it may be impossible to rouse the patient. The specific opioid antagonist naloxone should be given in such circumstances, 0.2–0.4 mg intravenously usually being sufficient, though larger and frequent doses may be necessary occasionally. Naloxone is more quickly eliminated than morphine (and therefore diamorphine) and it is possible to reverse respiratory depression only to have it recur later.

Diamorphine does not have marked cardiovascular effects if hypoxia and hypercarbia are avoided. Most opioids cause a degree of vasodilatation and, in high doses, myocardial depression. Clinically these are only likely to appear if there are other precipitating factors such as dehydration, incipient shock, etc.

Apart from the deleterious side-effects of diamorphine, there are some rather more desirable ones, such as sedation and tranquillity.

Naloxone is the specific antagonist to morphine and to most other opioids. Its use in respiratory depression has been described above, but it will reverse almost all the pharmacological effects of diamorphine. However, its use should be reserved for clinically obvious respiratory depression, especially when accompanied by deep sedation. This is because it will also reverse any analgesia that has been achieved, and the patient may experience severe pain for which there is no treatment, except by less effective non-opioid drugs.

Naloxone differs from diamorphine in its pharmacokinetics and it is possible to reverse the opioid effects only to have them return after 1 to 2 hours. Occasionally it is necessary to have a continuous infusion of the drug until normal respiratory control is achieved. Naloxone is available as 0.4 mg in 1 ml and 0.02 mg in 1 ml for neonates.

Respiratory depression due to diamorphine given in clinical doses is uncommon but may occur in sensitive patients or postoperatively if the drug has been given as a premedication or as an analgesic during anaesthesia. It should respond to quite small doses of naloxone, e.g., 0.1 mg IV, and the dosage should be titrated to the patient's response.

Diamorphine in postoperative pain

There is a general concensus that postoperative pain is badly treated in the majority of surgical units. This probably relates to the need for considerably more time and effort to be spent by the medical and nursing staff when the analgesia requires more than the simple prescription of an opioid p.r.n.

Nevertheless the institution of alternative regimes can be successful provided the clinicians and nurses are aware of the basic principles and there is agreement between the anaesthetic and surgical staff. In the early postoperative period, the residual effects of the anaesthetic must be allowed for.

The alternatives for postoperative pain relief are the following:

1. Use of the conventional intramuscular route. For this to be effective it is necessary for the initial dose to be carefully monitored both in regard to efficacy and side-effects. Diamorphine 5 mg is the standard dose but this should be reduced to 2.5 mg in the elderly. The patient should be questioned 30 minutes after the injection to assess the analgesia, the degree of sedation, and the presence or absence of respiratory depression as evidenced by a slow rate of breathing. This will act as a useful guide to subsequent dosage. The time course of the analgesia should also be noted so that an appropriate interval for repeat injections can be calculated. The great variation between individuals cannot be overemphasised and the frequency of injection may vary from 2 to 8 hours.

2. Use of a combined intravenous and intramuscular regime. A slow intravenous injection of diamorphine (2 mg/min) is given until the patient's pain is relieved. When the analgesia wears off, the same dose may be given intramuscularly, the interval depending upon the duration of analgesia.

3. Use of a continuous infusion of diamorphine. This should only be used if there is adequate supervision and monitoring and is generally only suitable for intensive care or high-dependancy units. Dosage is calculated from an initial intravenous injection given at 2 mg/min until analgesia is obtained. 25% of this dose is then infused hourly.

4. The use of a patient-controlled device. The added safety of self-administration allows these devices to be used in the ordinary postoperative ward.

5. Epidural diamorphine, which is fully described in Chapter 6 (see page 82). The most effective method is to infuse epidurally a combination of local anaesthetic and diamorphine. The infusion of two drugs (local anaesthetic and opioid) each with a quite different mode of action, gives very effective analgesia without the problem of overdosage (Hjortsø et al., 1986).

Diamorphine in pain relief in labour

Diamorphine is popular as an analgesic in labour and together with pethidine provides the commonest method of pain relief. While labour can occur with little or no pain, it may also be the most painful event in the life of a mother, particularly in her first delivery. The best results will undoubtedly be obtained when all the methods of pain relief have been discussed during the antenatal period and *her* choice has been fully considered.

Because of the severity of pain and the youth of the mothers, it is common practice to use diamorphine in rather higher dosage than in other indications, the standard intramuscular dose being 10 mg. The first dose should be given when labour is firmly established and the mother is requiring relief.

The duration of analgesia is relatively easy to assess as the uterine contractions are occurring at regular intervals.

Diamorphine, like all opioids, crosses the placenta with ease and will affect the foetal brain. It is usual therefore to try and avoid injections during the second stage of labour.

The important side-effects of diamorphine in labour are as follows:

1. The long delay caused in gastric emptying which allows the collection of large amounts of gastric fluid. This is of importance if general anaesthesia becomes necessary in an emergency. It is common therefore to restrict or prohibit oral food or fluid, an intravenous infusion being used to maintain fluid intake. Antacids given at regular intervals throughout labour are used to maintain a high pH in the stomach. If it is suspected that there is a significant amount of fluid in the stomach, a stomach tube should be passed before general anaesthesia is induced. Alternatively apomorphine (1–3 mg IV) can be given to induce emesis. Metoclopramide, to enhance gastric emptying, is relatively ineffective in the presence of opioid.
2. Nausea and vomiting.
3. Respiratory depression in the neonate. In units with appropriate facilities for the assessment and treatment of babies, this is of relatively minor importance as the administration of naloxone (0.01–0.02 mg IV) to the neonate is highly effective.

Conclusion

Although opioids in general, and diamorphine in particular, have been used to treat acute pain for a very long time, there is little doubt that their effectiveness could be greatly increased in hospital practice. This can be achieved by closer attention to the prescription and administration of these drugs, and to the monitoring of their effects, both in regard to analgesia and side-effects. Both the medical and nursing staff should understand the advantages and limitations of opioids, and particularly the varying needs of individual patients when the dosage is determined.

References

Evans, J. M., McCarthy, J., Rosen, M. and Hogg, M. I. J., (1978), 'Apparatus for patient-controlled administration of intravenous narcotics during labour', *Lancet*, **i**, 17.

Harmer, M., Rosen, M. and Vickers, M. D., (1985), *Patient-controlled Analgesia*, (Oxford, Blackwell Scientific Publications).

Hjortsø, N-C., Lund, C., Mogensen, T., Bigler, D. and Kehlet, H., (1986), 'Epidural morphine improves pain relief and maintains sensory analgesia during continuous epidural bupivacaine after abdominal surgery', *Anesthesia and Analgesia*, **65**, 1,033.

Kaiko, R. F., Wallenstein, S. L., Rogers, A. G., Grabinski, P. Y. and Houde, R. W., (1981), 'Analgesic and mood effects of heroin and morphine in cancer patients with postoperative pain', *New England Journal of Medicine*, **804**, 1,501.

Levine, M. N., Sackett, D. L. and Bush, H., (1966), 'Heroin vs morphine for cancer pain?', *Archives of Internal Medicine*, **146**, 353.

Macdonald, H. R., Muir, A. L., Rees, R. A., Lawrie, D. M., Burton, J. L. and Donald, K. W., (1967), 'Circulatory effects of heroin in patients with myocardial infarction', *Lancet*, **i**, 1,070.

Mather, L. E. and Phillips, G. D., (1986), 'Opioids and adjuvants: principles of use', in *Acute Pain Management*, Cousins, M. J. and Mather, L. E. (eds), (Melbourne, Churchill Livingstone, p. 77).

Mather, L. E., Lindop, M. J. and Tucker, G. T., (1975), 'Pethidine revisited: plasma concentration and effect after intramuscular injection', *British Journal of Anaesthesia*, **47**, 1,269.

Nimmo, W. S., Heading, R. C., Wilson, J., Tothill, P. and Prescott, L. F., (1975), 'Inhibition of gastric emptying and drug absorption by narcotic analgesics', *British Journal of Clinical Pharmacology*, **2**, 509.

Scott, M. E. and Orr, R., (1969), 'Effects of diamorphine, methadone, morphine and pentazocine in patients with suspected acute myocardial infarction', *Lancet*, **i**, 1,065.

DEREK DOYLE, OBE, FRCSE, FRCPE, FRCGP

5 Opioid therapy in terminal cancer

The opioids, morphine and diamorphine in particular, remain unchallenged as the ultimate analgesics for patients with the pains of far-advanced cancer. They are the yardstick against which all others are measured. In spite of being available in many convenient formulations, they are often withheld unnecessarily or prescribed inappropriately when experience shows that they are necessary in approximately 60% of these patients and are capable, either alone or in combination, of controlling the pain in 95% of them.

Cancer pain

Eight different types of pain may be encountered in patients with cancer, some of which are amenable to a specific therapy which may be effective, either alone or when combined with an opioid.

1. Pain due to bone secondaries. This would initially merit palliative radiotherapy, preferably with adjuvant prostaglandin biosynthetase inhibitors, and is likely to be effective after two or three weeks. Opioids are nearly always required eventually.

2. Nerve entrapment pain. This is caused by vertebral collapse, tumour compression or postoperative or postradiation fibrosis and is localised to adjacent dermatomes. It will usually respond to low-dose oral steroids, but in about 5% of such patients, a neurolytic procedure, for example with 5% phenol in glycerin given intrathecally, will be necessary.

3. Visceral pain in liver, spleen or kidney caused by the stretching of

the capsule as the organ is infiltrated by secondaries. Occasionally, when haemorrhage occurs in the secondary deposit, the pain may be acute and mimic an abdominal emergency. Visceral pain usually necessitates an opioid, but may also benefit from an adjuvant steroid.

4. Soft-tissue pain, which is often associated with adenopathy in thorax, abdomen or pelvis, may initially respond to a medium-strength analgesic but usually requires a potent opioid eventually.

5. Colic pain, no different in character from colic due to any other pathology, is surprisingly uncommon in terminally-ill patients, but is still occasionally seen and should be treated with anti-spasmodics.

6. Headache, associated with raised intercranial pressure from cerebral oedema produced by primary or secondary cerebral tumours. Relief often follows the reduction of oedema with dexamethasone and patients rarely benefit from opioids.

7. Joint pain, which is no different in cause or character from that encountered with any of the arthritidies. Opioids are rarely called for, and relief usually follows the prescription of a non-steroidal anti-inflammatory drug (NSAID).

8. Dysaesthesia, usually responsive to clonidine, sodium valproate or tricyclic anti-depressants, is rarely helped by opioids.

It is not uncommon for patients to have three or four different kinds of pain at the one time and to require different medication for each. For example, there may be pain from bone secondaries, right hypochondrial pain from stretching the liver capsule, vague low-back pain from para-aortic nodes or constipation, headache from cerebral metastases and dysaesthesia in a lymphoedematous arm. It is important to remember that in terminally-ill cancer patients, 25% of pain or discomfort is not directly due to the cancer. For example, there may be constipation, bed sores, chronic osteoarthritis, osteoporosis or postradiation colitis, to name but a few.

Analgesic management

The analgesic 'ladder'

General practitioners should have no hesitation in prescribing a strong opioid when it is called for. It is logical, however, to begin with non-opioid analgesic (usually a NSAID), and maintain the patient on that so long as it controls the pain without adverse effects. If this becomes ineffective, the treatment should be changed to a weak opioid, such as codeine, dex-

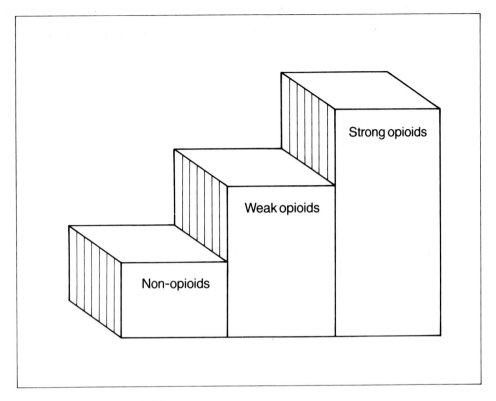

Fig. 5.1 The analgesic 'ladder'.

tropropoxyphene, dihydrocodeine, dipipanone or one of the agonist/ antagonist opioid drugs such as buprenorphine (see Fig. 5.1).

When that drug either fails to control the pain or adverse effects appear, the prescription must then be changed to a strong opioid. Knowledge of the approximate analgesic equivalent of different drugs will enable this to be done without any break in analgesia (see Fig. 5.2).

For example, a patient on dipipanone and cyclizine (Diconal), 20 mg 6-hourly, is on the equivalent of 40 mg oral morphine daily. If this dose is not controlling the pain, he should be changed to oral morphine solution, 60 mg daily, given as 10 mg every 4 hours.

If the patient has not been on an escalating analgesic regimen and it is decided to start with a strong opioid, a good rule is to give oral morphine solution, 10 mg every 4 hours. The very frail or elderly patient would be started on 5 mg or even 2.5 mg. The earlier the patient is started on the opioid the slower will increments be needed. More important, however, is that the doctor should have the confidence to build up the dose to that which controls the pain. The author, like all in full-time terminal care, has seen hundreds of patients whose pain is perfectly controlled on doses as

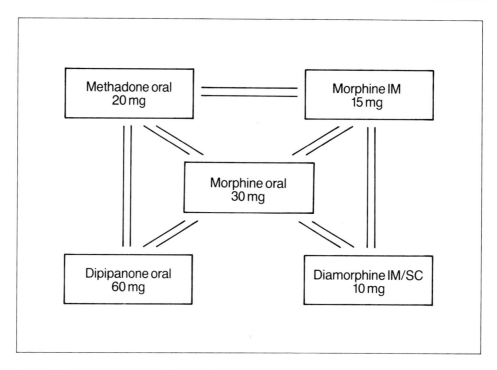

Fig. 5.2 Terminal care: opioid equivalents.

low as 10 mg 4-hourly, but equally, has seen young patients, remarkably mobile and active, on doses of 300 mg (or even higher) 4-hourly. *High dosage is not synonymous with deep sedation and inability to behave normally.*

This analgesic ladder makes good pharmacological sense; it is simple to follow and it is now internationally accepted and recommended. (World Health Organization, *Cancer Pain Relief*, 1986.)

Analgesic doses in terminal cancer

It may be stated categorically that the correct dose of a strong opioid for any individual patient is that which controls the pain.

Many patients are forced to endure pain because of a doctor's reluctance to prescribe an adequate dose for fear of respiratory depression. There should never be any hesitation, however, in increasing the dose until the pain is controlled because pain is the physiological antagonist to the central suppressant effects of the opioids.

Conversely it is important to remember that reduction in pain achieved by other means (e.g., by neurolytic procedure or radiotherapy) will remove the body's physiological antagonist. This may lead to evidence of opioid toxicity such as depression of respiration, pinpoint pupils, coma, etc.

Morphine and diamorphine

Provided equi-analgesic doses are employed, there is little to choose between these two drugs, contrary to what was often thought and taught.

The major advantage of diamorphine over morphine is its greater water solubility, making it the drug of choice for injections, because large volumes can be avoided. When injected, diamorphine acts more quickly than morphine, due to its greater lipid solubility.

For oral administration morphine may be preferable to diamorphine because, being a less potent analgesic, its dose in solution can more easily be titrated to the patient's need. In solution, diamorphine undergoes hydrolysis to 6-O-acetylmorphine and then slowly to morphine itself. However, acetylmorphine is equipotent with diamorphine and no loss of analgesia occurs until it is hydrolysed to morphine, which may take several weeks (see page 8).

Oral administration

Morphine solution

Morphine may be given as one of the following:

    (a) a solution of the sulphate or hydrochloride salt;

    (b) a controlled-release tablet;

    (c) a buccal tablet.

Diamorphine solution

Diamorphine may be given as one of the following:

    (a) a solution of the hydrochloride salt;

    (b) a sub-lingual tablet.

The solutions are simply morphine or diamorphine dissolved in water, chloroform water (acting as a preservative) or sodium metabisulphite (200 parts per million), the latter being reported as no more palatable or acceptable to the patient, but equally efficacious (see also Chapter 1, page 12).

The prescription should be for the desired dose of morphine or diamorphine, dissolved in 10 ml of the solvent. A useful starting dose of morphine is 10 mg. It should be given on a regular 4-hourly basis and never 'p.r.n.'.

If pain persists, the dose is increased until control is achieved. Logical as it seems to increase the frequency of administration rather than increasing the dose, this soon leads to a patient taking the solution every 2 or 3 hours (*ad lib*) and places an unnecessary and unacceptable responsibility on the patient or his relatives.

Until control is achieved and maintained for 4 or 5 days, the night dose given at 2 a.m. should not be omitted. Only rarely will the patient complain about being wakened for its administration. Thereafter it is usually possible to give a double dose at 10 p.m. and the next dose at 6 a.m., presumably because of the slower metabolic rate at night.

Brompton's mixture ('cocktail')
Various formularies list several different morphine or diamorphine mixtures containing such additions as alcohol, cocaine and chlorpromazine, almost all of which at one time or another have gone under the name 'Brompton's mixture' (see page 12).

It must be stated that not only is this confusing and quite unscientific, but there is no evidence whatsoever that these formulations have any advantage over a simple morphine-in-water solution. Alcohol produces a most unpleasant 'bite' which distresses the patient with candidosis. Cocaine has been shown to have no analgesic properties and its stimulant effect is not called for. An added phenothiazine produces unacceptable sedation and, in the long term, unwanted extra-pyramidal effects. Its antiemetic properties will not be needed after the first few days and there are more preferable antiemetics available. The term, and the formulation of, 'Brompton's mixture' should now be relegated to the books of medical history.

Controlled-release morphine tablets
These are available in strengths of 10 mg, 30 mg, 60 mg and 100 mg, formulated to achieve a peak plasma concentration after 4 hours and to maintain it for 8 to 12 hours. Thus, they should be taken 12-hourly but *never* on a p.r.n. basis. When a patient suffers pain breakthrough and requires immediate analgesia, it is unscientific to advise him to take a tablet which will not achieve analgesia for 4 hours. Similarly, when pain is not controlled on controlled-release morphine tablets, or breaks through before the next dose is due, it is illogical to increase the frequency of administration with such a formulation. A higher dose of tablet is required, still given on a 12-hourly basis.

Patients should not be started on c.r.m. tablets until the total daily requirements of morphine have been ascertained using oral morphine solution for at least 5 to 7 days. The dose is calculated by dividing the 24-hour requirement by two and giving it 12-hourly. For example, a patient whose pain has come under control on oral morphine solution 10 mg every 4 hours (i.e., 60 mg in 24 hours) may find it more acceptable to take c.r.m. tablets 30 mg 12-hourly. A patient on oral morphine solution of 200 mg every 4 hours (i.e., 1200 mg in 24 hours) will require tablets 600 mg every 12 hours.

Some doctors use these tablets as a means of prescribing morphine without having to tell the patient he is on an opioid, with all the public misunderstanding and fears about these drugs. This practice is to be condemned. Terminally-ill patients have a right to know exactly what they are receiving and why. They should always be given truthful explanations about all details of their illness, its treatment and its prognosis.

Buccal morphine tablets

These controlled-release tablets are still being developed, but may prove useful because they avoid first-pass metabolism in the liver. As a result, satisfactory plasma concentrations are said to be more quickly achieved.

Rectal administration

Morphine is available in suppository form, 15 mg, and 30 mg, though any strength can be made on request in the pharmacy.

The suppository appears to be capable of achieving equivalent plasma levels and analgesia as by the oral route, but their use is obviously limited by patient acceptance, the regularity of bowel evacuation, the use and types of laxatives and the presence of rectal pathology. Morphine suppositories should be given 4-hourly. (See also Chapter 1, page 12.)

Parenteral administration

Subcutaneous injection

As already stated, the main advantage of diamorphine is its greater water-solubility, making it the drug of choice for injection. This is especially so when any large doses are being injected. 1·0 gm of diamorphine can be dissolved in only 1·6 ml of water, whereas 21 ml of water are required for 1·0 gm of morphine sulphate, and 24 ml of water for 1·0 gm of morphine hydrochloride. Though saline can be used as the solvent, it is preferable, for reasons of hypertonicity, to use water when strengths of greater than 500 mg of diamorphine are being used. Diamorphine may be given subcutaneously by intermittent injection or continuous infusion. With the former the dose is one-third of the dose of oral morphine being given. For example, a patient on oral morphine solution, 30 mg every 4 hours, who is considered, for one reason or another, to need diamorphine injections, will require 10 mg, subcutaneously, every 4 hours round the clock. A continuous subcutaneous infusion, delivered by a compact battery-operated syringe driver/pump, obviates the need for 4-hourly injections, the needle being left *in situ* for about 4 days and the giving-set changed every 14 days. The syringe requires refilling once daily.

The 24-hour requirements of diamorphine, using this method, are calculated either from the total oral morphine, or the intermittent subcutaneous diamorphine requirements of the previous days. For example, a patient on oral morphine solution of 60 mg every 4 hours (360 mg in 24 hours), would require 120 mg diamorphine. The patient previously on, for example, 20 mg diamorphine, subcutaneously, every 4 hours, will also require 120 mg dissolved in 10 ml of sterile water.

The compatibility of drugs, particularly antiemetics, with the injectable solution of diamorphine administered subcutaneously via a syringe driver, varies considerably (see also page 10). If mixtures are to be used, it should be for the shortest possible time, and the syringe should be recharged daily if possible.

It must be noted that sterile inflammatory skin reactions may occur at the site of injection related, not only to the additive, but also to the strength of diamorphine injected. The higher the dose, the greater the likelihood of a reaction. When they occur, the only course of action is to change to an alternative site. If they persist, the patient must be put back on to 4-hourly injections.

Useful as this method of injection undoubtedly is, the indications for it are limited. While in domiciliary terminal care its advantages are obvious, in hospital practice the only advantage is for the emaciated patient with poor injection sites. There is no reason to think that a continuous subcutaneous infusion achieves and maintains plasma levels better than intermittent injections because there is the problem that uptake may be poor from subcutaneous tissues in the cachectic patient.

Intravenous infusion or injection of diamorphine
Tolerance to the opioids appears to develop more rapidly when they are given intravenously than when given subcutaneously or intramuscularly. The use of an intravenous injection is justifiable for the control of sudden, severe pain provided appropriate measures are taken to prevent its recurrence. The only justification for continuous intravenous infusion in terminal care is the patient who is already receiving intravenous fluid for some other reason, or who is so grossly emaciated that injection sites are at a premium.

Epidural administration
Constipation is an unavoidable and troublesome side-effect of the opioids. The higher the dose of the opioid, the greater the problem of constipation, and the more laxatives that are required. Any measure which will enable pain to be controlled with the smallest possible dose of opioid merits consideration. When an opioid is introduced directly into the central nervous system, a much smaller dose is required because it acts directly on the opioid receptors and, in particular, on the endorphin-secreting cells of the substantia gelatinosa of the spinal cord. In consequence of the lower dose, there is less constipation and, in theory, more predictable efficacy leads to increased patient-acceptance and compliance.

This method of opioid administration necessitates a high level of technical skill in introducing a plastic catheter (and possibly a reservoir), and the use of sterile, pyrogen and preservative-free drug. A fine plastic catheter is introduced into the epidural space at the level of the dermatome with most pain, and brought round to the front of the abdomen in a subcutaneous tunnel. The end of the catheter may be brought out through the skin of the anterior abdominal wall and fitted with a disposable bacterial filter. The required dose of opioid is injected intermittently, through the filter, with the necessary antiseptic precautions. Alternatively, a small specially-designed reservoir can be attached to the end of the catheter and implanted immediately beneath the skin of the anterior abdominal wall. The reservoir slowly infuses the drug into the epidural space. It is refilled at intervals by inserting a needle through the skin and injecting fresh drug.

Ideal as the route and the method may sound, in practice there are often problems. The catheter tip, though its position will have been checked radiologically at the time of insertion, may migrate out of the epidural space. The catheter itself may block or be a route for the entry of infection. The weight of the bacterial filter may kink the catheter, causing it to crack, and for this reason the newer subcutaneous reservoir may have decided advantages.

Interestingly, the respiratory depressant effect of the opioid is antagonised by naloxone, while the analgesia persists.

The epidural route has a place in the care of terminally-ill cancer patients whose pain is otherwise difficult to control, and in whom constipation is a major problem. It is not first-line treatment.

Adverse effects of opioids

Nausea and vomiting

Nausea may be encountered in the first 4 to 7 days in about 30% of patients on oral morphine solution, and in no more than 10% of patients starting on c.r.m. tablets. Thereafter, unless the dose is rapidly increased, it tends to disappear and, contrary to long-held belief, vomiting is uncommon with these drugs.

An antiemetic may be needed, but should not be prescribed routinely. There seems little to choose between the different antiemetics. The author's preference is either haloperidol 1.5 to 2.5 mg daily or metoclopramide 10 mg t.i.d. for the first few days.

It should be noted that, at higher doses, morphine appears to block the gastric-emptying effects of metoclopramide. There is no benefit in routinely prescribing phenothiazines, such as chlorpromazine or prochlorperazine, whose sedative effects are usually unacceptable to these patients.

Sedation

Drowsiness also tends to pass off within a few days. However, the patient, freed from pain, bored and not stimulated, can develop inactivity drowsiness. The patient should be reassured on this point, and he or she should not be taken off the drug.

The question of driving motor vehicles occasionally arises in patients who are fully active and achieving full pain control on the opioids. The taking of long-term opioids under strict medical supervision is not in itself an absolute contra-indication to driving. Clearly the doctor has the same responsibility as for any patient suffering a physical handicap, or on drugs likely to impair concentration, slow responses or diminish alertness. The wisest course is obviously to advise the patient not to drive. For further advice, the doctor in Britain may contact the Medical Advisory Branch at the Driver and Vehicle Licensing Centre, Swansea SA1 1TU, telephone Swansea (0792) 42731.

Confusion, dizziness and dysphoria

These may all occur in older patients who should accordingly be forewarned. Occasionally the dose will need to be reduced and then built up again more gradually. It is rare for patients to become psychotic on these drugs, though sometimes they do. Should it occur, the opioid will have to be discontinued, or the dose reduced and the patient put onto a phenothiazine. Contrary to what is often expected, long-term use of the opioids may lead to dysphoria rather than euphoria and this may be corrected with a tricyclic anti-depressant.

Constipation and urinary retention

It cannot be overstated that, unless there is some pre-existing pathology producing diarrhoea or steatorrhoea, all patients become constipated on the opioids, and the use of an appropriate laxative is mandatory. The management and correction of constipation are often more difficult than the control of pain and require just as much skill and attention to detail.

Urinary retention is uncommon, but should it occur, continuous bladder drainage may be necessary. It is sometimes associated with epidural opioids.

Interaction with other drugs

Agonist/antagonist

Drugs such as buprenorphine, meptazinol and pentazocine compete with opioid agonists for receptor sites. They should therefore not be prescribed concurrently with the pure agonists morphine and diamorphine. Inadvertent use of the two competitive groups is a common cause of poor pain control.

There should not be any breakthrough pain in the transition from an agonist/antagonist to a pure agonist because the latter will bind to the receptors that are newly vacated by the former.

Benzodiazepines

In terminal care, there are indications for benzodiazepines such as lorazepam for panic attacks, diazepam for muscle relaxation and temazepam for night sedation. There are no pharmacological reasons why these drugs cannot be given alongside the opioids provided it is remembered that the sedative effect may be more marked, and unacceptable to the patient.

Phenothiazines

These drugs do not potentiate morphine or diamorphine. They are potent sedatives and it is most unusual for a terminally-ill patient either to ask for, or to accept, daytime sedation. More commonly this is requested by the relatives, or suggested by the doctor, to ease the responsibility of listening to and talking to the patient. Because of the sedative effect of the phenothiazines there is no justification for their routine inclusion in an oral morphine solution. For ill-understood reasons, the higher the dose of the opioid being used, the higher the dose required of the benzodiazepine or the phenothiazine. One encounters the occasional patient on 600–1000 mg daily of morphine and taking 20–30 mg or more of diazepam without any evidence of sedation.

Failure with the opioids

Extremely useful though the opioids are, they are not panaceas. Pain control demands the most scrupulous attention to every detail of the patient's condition, not least his many other physical, emotional, social and spiritual needs. Nevertheless, experience suggests that there are many patients in whom the opioids are the most appropriate analgesics, but who do not achieve optimal benefit. Some reasons for this are as follows:

1. Opioids are often under-prescribed until the final days of life because of the unnecessary fear that:
   (a) tolerance will rapidly develop, and the doctor will have to prescribe higher doses than those with which he is familiar;

(b) addiction will be a problem;

(c) there will be depression of respiration;

(d) the patient may use the drug for suicide;

(e) the relatives may use the drug for euthanasia;

(f) the opioid will be stolen by an addict.

Experience shows that the earlier the opioid is prescribed, the more gradual the increments, the fewer the adverse effects (excepting constipation), and the greater the chance that the dose may actually be reduced.

2. Agonists/antagonists are given concurrently.

3. Neurolytic procedures are not employed, exclusive hope being placed in the opioids. Nerve blocks can be extremely useful in:

(a) unilateral trunk pain restricted to adjacent dermatomes;

(b) carcinoma of pancreas infiltrating the L1 vertebra;

(c) perineal pain, whether from carcinoma of the prostate, rectum or genito-urinary tract;

(d) tumours of the head and neck provided access to the Gasserian ganglion or the main branches of the trigeminal nerve is possible.

Alcohol hypophysectomy should be considered for generalised pain, secondary to such hormone-sensitive tumours as breast and prostate.

Within an hour or so of a successful neurolytic procedure, the pain may be so reduced as to remove its physiological antagonism to the opioids, resulting in immediate, and potentially catastrophic, depression of respiration. For this reason such patients must be monitored after the procedure, and the doctor should be prepared to reduce the maintenance opioid dose appropriately.

4. Inadequate attention is paid to insomnia which, though often due to poorly-controlled pain, is more frequently secondary to unventilated or unresolved fears. If it can be demonstrated that insomnia is due to pain, the opioid regime can be changed accordingly by giving a larger dose at 10 p.m. If it is not due to pain, the doctor should not automatically prescribe a short-acting benzodiazepine until every opportunity has been given for the patient to express his fears, and honest explanations have been given about his condition, both to him and each principal member of the family, perhaps as a group.

5. Opioid absorption may be impaired as with gastric pathology, malabsorption syndrome, oedema of the gut, or persistent vomiting from whatever cause.

6. Renal function, rather than hepatic function, has not been asses-sed before beginning the opioids. There is accumulating evidence that impaired renal function necessitates lower opioid doses. It follows that in any patient who is becoming drowsy, the doctor must assess whether it is due to progress of the disease (possibly with cerebral metastases), excessive sedation with other drugs, more opioid than is required for pain control, or impaired excretion of the opioid and its metabolites, because of failing renal function.

Conclusion

It is as wrong to use opioids indiscriminately as it is to withhold them without good reason. They remain the most useful analgesics we possess for terminal care but, as with all drugs, the best results only follow skilled assessment, attention to fine detail, titration of the dose against the patient's needs, responsiveness to patient compliance and acceptance, and regular consultation with nursing colleagues. It should be possible to achieve pain control without undue sedation or other unacceptable side-effects in not less than 95% of patients dying from carcinoma.

References

Twycross, R. G. and Lack, S. A., (1983), 'Symptom control in far advanced cancer', in *Pain Relief*, (London, Pitman).

Twycross, R. G. and Lack, S. A., (1984), *Therapeutics in Terminal Cancer*, (London, Pitman).

Doyle, D., (1984), *Palliative Care: the management of far advanced illness*, (London: Croom Helm).

Doyle, D., (1987), *Domiciliary Terminal Care*, (Edinburgh, Churchill Livingstone).

Twycross, R. G., (1984), *Clinics in Oncology: pain relief in cancer*, **3**, (No. 1), (London, Saunders).

Wall, P. D. and Melsacz, R., (1984), *Textbook of Pain*, (Edinburgh, Churchill Livingstone).

Hanks, G. W. and Hoskin, P. J., (1987), 'Opioid analgesics in the management of pain in patients with cancer', *Palliative Medicine*, **1**, (No.1), 1–25

Cherry, D. A. and Gourlay, G. K., (1987), 'The spinal administration of opioids in the treatment of acute and chronic pain: bolus doses, continuous infusion, intraventricular administration and implanted drug delivery systems', *Palliative Medicine*, **1**, (No.2), 89–106.

LEON KAUFMAN, MD, FFARCS

6 Intraspinal diamorphine: epidural and intrathecal

In 1976, Yaksh and Rudy demonstrated that intrathecal opioids produced naloxone-reversible analgesia in animals. This study prompted the introduction of intrathecal morphine (0.5–1 mg) by Wang *et al.*, 1979, for pain relief in inoperable carcinoma. In 1976, Martin *et al.* had propounded the concept that there were multi-receptor sites to explain some of the actions of opioids. For example, the μ-receptor is associated with analgesia, respiratory depression and small pupils, while the α-receptor is associated with the psychological effects.

Sensory afferent nerve fibres of peripheral nerves terminate in the dorsal horn of the spinal cord, in lamina II, of the substantia gelatinosa, where there are high concentrations of opioid receptors, endorphins and substance P. Opioids inhibit the release of substance P and appear to be particularly effective in suppressing the pain associated with deep sensation which is transmitted in peripheral nerves by C-fibres. They are less effective in suppressing the acute pain of surgery which is transmitted largely by A-delta-fibres. These are readily blocked by local anaesthetics.

Morphine is active at μ-receptor sites which are present in the cerebral cortex, the periaquaductal grey region in the brain, and in the dorsal horn. There are ϰ-receptors in the spinal cord where dynorphins are believed to be the transmitter. From experimental studies it now appears there are both μ-1 and μ-2 sites, the former associated with analgesia and the latter with respiratory depression. Morphine, diamorphine, pethidine and fentanyl are agonists at μ-receptors, while pentazocine, nalbuphine and butorphanol have antagonist properties at μ-sites and agonist actions at ϰ-sites.

These studies, although intensely stimulating, appear to confuse the clinician as to their significance. The characteristics and principles of action of spinal opioids have been reviewed by Yaksh, 1981, while Martin,

1984, has produced an up-to-date account of the detailed pharmacology of opioids.

Although the mode of action of spinal opioids is still subject to debate, what is not disputed is their efficacy in the suppression of pain. The concept of opioids having a localized action is not entirely new. Alexander Wood, who is credited with being the first to use the syringe for medical purposes, injected painful areas with morphine as long ago as 1853, while Feldberg in 1959 was experimenting with the direct injection of drugs into the cerebral ventricles. It seemed logical to place drugs in small quantities as near as possible to receptor sites along the spinal cord. Intraspinal injection may be made either into the epidural space or into the subarachnoid (intrathecal) space to avoid giving larger doses intramuscularly which are effective only after systemic absorption.

The onset and duration of action appears to be related to the lipid partition coefficient of the opioid. Morphine, having a low solubility in lipid, is slow in onset but prolonged in duration. Diamorphine, fentanyl and pethidine are much more lipid soluble and can rapidly cross tissue barriers such as the dura mater and diffuse through the nerve membranes in the spinal cord, to reach the receptor sites. A drug which is given epidurally has first to penetrate the dura, whereas, if the agent is given intrathecally, there is no dura to cross, and the receptor site is reached rapidly even with morphine. While high-lipid solubility allows rapid access when given epidurally, it also allows a quicker release from receptors, explaining the shorter duration.

The attraction of intraspinal opioids for pain relief is that a small dose can be administered near to its site of action, resulting in reversible analgesia, but affecting only painful sensory inputs. The motor nerves and other sensory modalities are unaffected, in contrast to the actions of local anaesthetics, and no anaesthesia or motor paralysis will develop. Similarly, hypotension does not ensue, as opioids do not suppress activity of the autonomic nerves. The intraspinal route thus obviates the need for large parenteral doses which may have effects on other organs, particularly the brain. Intraspinal opioids have potential for treatment of chronic pain without involving prolonged or permanent nerve blockade, as occurs with intrathecal phenol whose effects may be irreversible.

Choice of drugs

Many opioids have been given intraspinally for the relief of postoperative pain, including morphine, pethidine, methadone, fentanyl and buprenorphine.

The author's personal choice of diamorphine was influenced by its effectiveness in the rapid relief of pain in patients with inoperable carcinoma, with analgesia lasting for up to 48 hours. Diamorphine is lipophilic, readily crosses membranes and is converted to monoacetyl morphine and morphine at the site of action. It is easy to sterilise, the freeze-dried preparation being readily autoclavable without loss of potency.

Diamorphine is considered to be safer than morphine for intrathecal and epidural use, because of its greater lipophilicity and shorter half-life. These factors are of great importance because the concentrations in the cerebrospinal fluid (CSF) of diamorphine or morphine, given intrathecally, are 4000 times greater than that seen following intravenous morphine, 1 mg/kg (Moore et al., 1984). Because of its low lipid solubility, morphine remains in the CSF much longer than diamorphine, and this allows it to spread cephalad and occasionally cause respiratory depression. There have been numerous reports of delayed respiratory depression, or apnoea, following intrathecal morphine, in contrast to the absence of adverse comment on the use of diamorphine, although it must be conceded that the latter drug has been less frequently used. Kotob et al., 1986, showed that the absorption of diamorphine from the subarachnoid space occurred more rapidly than with morphine, their elimination half-lives from the CSF being 43 minutes and 73 minutes respectively. Diamorphine was rapidly converted in the plasma to morphine, and the peak plasma concentration of morphine, derived from diamorphine, was higher than 47.8 nmol/l and reached that point more rapidly (10 mins) than did morphine (8.2 nmol/l and 216 mins), following the intrathecal injection of 1 mg of both drugs.

It would appear that diamorphine is a safer drug as the onset of action and duration are shorter. Because of its high lipophilicity, diamorphine readily crosses membranes and delivers not only the drug itself, but its two active metabolites, monoacetyl morphine and morphine, to the site of action. On the other hand, morphine being less lipophilic, crosses membranes more slowly and therefore the onset is insidious and the duration of action prolonged and unpredictable. In addition morphine-6-glucuronide, one of the breakdown products of morphine, is 40 times more potent than morphine when injected intracerebrally in animals. This may be a factor in the prolonged action of the parent drug.

Indications

Intraoperative analgesia

Patients undergoing abdominal operations are usually induced with an intravenous hypnotic, such as thiopentone, followed by a muscle relaxant for intubation, and thereafter they are ventilated with nitrous oxide and oxygen, relaxation being maintained by incremental doses of muscle relaxants. The analgesic action of nitrous oxide may be supplemented with volatile agents or intravenous opioids, such as fentanyl or alfentanil. In some centres, patients receive very light levels of anaesthesia, while analgesia and muscular relaxation are provided by local anaesthetia given intrathecally or epidurally.

However, there have only been a few reports of the use of intrathecal diamorphine given specifically to produce analgesia at operation.

Intrathecal diamorphine

In the author's own series of 350 patients, 2.5–5 mg of diamorphine in 5–10 ml saline were administered intrathecally, following induction of anaesthesia, which was maintained with nitrous oxide and oxygen, intermittent increments of a muscle relaxant (atracurium) and, occasionally, with a volatile anaesthetic agent. The technique involved performing a lumbar puncture, preferably at L3–4 using a 22- or 25-gauge spinal needle. The solution was injected, without barbotage, over a period of not less than 1 minute, the needle being left *in situ* for at least a further minute to prevent possible seepage from the dural puncture. The duration of the surgical procedures varied from 3 to 8 hours for operations including anterior resection and abdominoperineal resection of the rectum. The use of intrathecal diamorphine provided excellent operative conditions without hypotension that could be attributable to anaesthesia. Explorative procedures in the upper abdomen sometimes caused transient increases in blood pressure which reverted to normal with cessation of the stimulus.

Intrathecal diamorphine is more effective than intravenous fentanyl in suppressing the hyperglycaemic and adrenocorticol response to surgical stimulation (see Figs 6.1, 6.2). Plasma cortisol levels were significantly less in patients given intrathecal diamorphine 90 minutes after skin incision and postoperatively for up to 6 hours. These effects may have contributed to the improved patient well-being in the postoperative period (Child and Kaufman, 1985). Intrathecal diamorphine also attenuated the usual rise in antidiurectic hormone in response to surgical stimulation for the duration of operation (Kaufman and Bailey, 1987) (see Fig. 6.3).

Epidural diamorphine

Diamorphine may be given epidurally to provide operative analgesia. This is less effective than by the intrathecal route. The main advantage of the epidural route is to provide postoperative analgesia by intermittent injection via an epidural catheter.

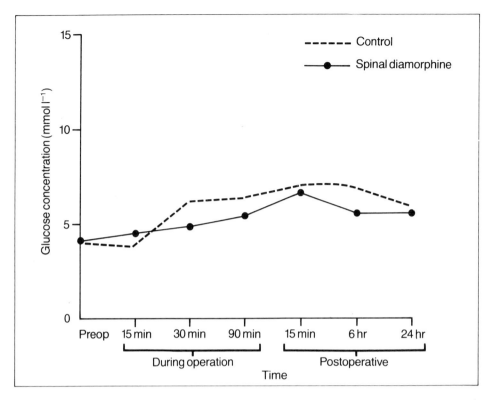

Fig. 6.1 Effect of intraoperative and postoperative diamorphine on plasma glucose.

Postoperative analgesia

Epidural diamorphine

Epidural diamorphine has been used to produce postoperative pain relief following a variety of surgical procedures. After thoracotomy and lower abdominal surgery, Jacobson *et al.*, 1983, administered 0.1 mg/kg in 10 ml saline and reported satisfactory results. The duration of pain relief was more prolonged when compared with intramuscular injections. However, Phillips *et al.*, 1984, reported less favourable results for post-thoracotomy cases using only 2 mg of diamorphine in 10 ml saline.

Epidural diamorphine has also been used for the postoperative management of patients undergoing partial or complete cystectomy. The operative procedure was undertaken under epidural analgesia with local anaesthetic agents and postoperative pain relief achieved with repeated doses of 2.5 mg of diamorphine in 10 ml saline via the same epidural catheter (Krapez, personal communication).

Watson *et al.*, 1984, reported impressive analgesia following lumbar laminectomy. An epidural catheter was positioned under direct vision at operation and 5 mg of diamorphine, given by this route, produced

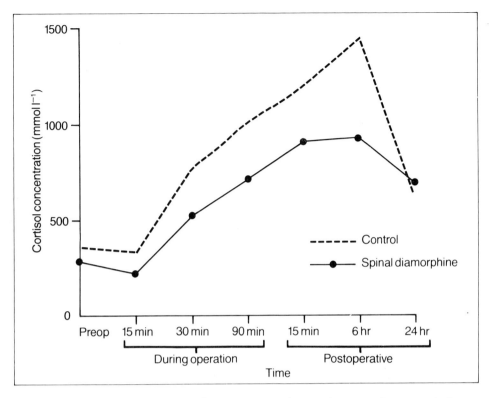

Fig. 6.2 Effect of intraoperative and postoperative diamorphine on plasma cortisol.

analgesia ranging from 185–560 minutes (median 360 mins).

Diamorphine has been administered by the caudal route (2.5 mg in 10 ml saline) to produce postoperative analgesia following haemorrhoidectomy. Diamorphine produced longer-lasting pain relief than 20 ml of 0.5% bupivacaine, 60% of the patients requiring no analgesia in the first postoperative 24-hours. Urinary retention only occurred in the bupivacaine group of patients (Bailey and Sangwan, 1986).

Intrathecal diamorphine

Intrathecal diamorphine was used successfully by Barron and Strong, 1984, for more than 900 patients undergoing total hip replacement, and for 150 patients having spinal surgery. For the former operation, the drug was administered by lumbar puncture, whereas in the latter group it was administered by the surgeon, under direct vision. The dose administered was within the range of 0.005–0.015 mg/kilo, but the total dose never exceeded 1 mg. There was no clinical evidence of respiratory depression in any of the patients, and 40% of them required no other postoperative analgesic. The use of naloxone was not required.

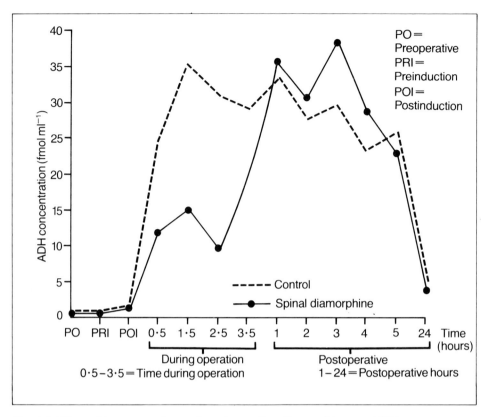

Fig. 6.3 Effect of intraoperative and postoperative diamorphine on ADH concentration.

Not only does intrathecal diamorphine provide intraoperative analgesia, as well as suppressing the endocrine response to surgery, it provides prolonged postoperative pain relief. In an analysis of the first 230 patients given intrathecal diamorphine in the author's personal series referred to above, the average duration of pain relief was 16 hours. Of these patients, 116 (50%) required no further analgesia in the first 24 hours, while 70 (30%) were pain-free beyond this time (see Fig. 6.4). Two patients had no postoperative narcotic analgesia whatsoever. This is in marked contrast to the use of intravenous opioids during major surgery. Postoperative analgesia was usually required within the first postoperative hour following the use of multiple doses of fentanyl during operation. Intravenous diamorphine (10 mg) resulted in analgesia for up to 4 hours postoperatively.

The dose of diamorphine administered intrathecally was approximately 0.5 mg/10 kg of body weight, and the volume of saline 1 ml/30 cm of patient height. Unfortunately, there appeared to be no direct relationship between the duration of analgesia and the patient's height, weight,

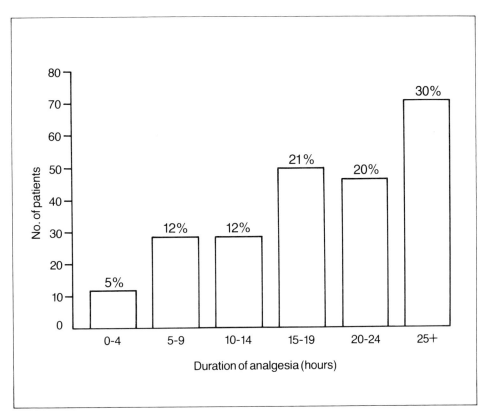

Fig. 6.4 Duration of analgesia.

the dose of drug, or the volume injected. Age appeared to be the only significant factor affecting the response, and therefore the dose should be markedly reduced in the elderly.

There are also physical factors which may influence the action of diamorphine in saline. The specific gravity of the solution may alter with temperature, while there is a wide variation for normal saline (0.9%) that is allowed by the BP assay limits (Williams, 1984). The solution may leak out through the dura puncture if too large a spinal needle is used, or if the patient strains soon after the solution is injected.

Spinal opioids have little effect upon pain from the wound, and patients who have a low tolerance to skin pain are more likely to complain of lack of analgesia. This was noted particularly in female patients. The use of neostigmine to antagonise muscle relaxants at the end of surgery may cause painful colicky contractions, despite the use of intravenous atropine.

The technique of intrathecal diamorphine is welcomed by the nursing staff who are able to move pain-free patients in the postoperative phase, while physiotherapy can be instituted without discomfort, encouraging patients to breathe deeply. Unfortunately improvement in respiratory function, as assessed by simple spirometeric tests, has been disappointing (Staren and Cullen, 1986).

Epidural bupivacaine and morphine

Epidural bupivacaine does not always provide complete postoperative pain relief and this prompted Hjortsø et al., 1986, to suggest that this might be remedied by introducing an opioid as well. It was found that the addition of morphine (0.5 mg/hr) to a continuous infusion of bupivacaine 0.5% (8 ml/hr) improved pain relief for at least 16 hours, and suggested that the combined use of the drugs could maintain analgesia for 2–4 days.

Intrathecal pethidine

Pethidine is usually prescribed for its analgesic action, but it also has a local anaesthetic affect. These attributes of the drug prompted Acalouschi et al., 1986, to use intrathecal pethidine for perineal surgery, 100 mg in 2 ml saline: this produced sensory blockade (S2–5) which was later followed by motor blockade. Cozain et al., 1986, reported similar results using 1 mg/kg of pethidine in 1 ml of 30% dextrose, given intrathecally to patients undergoing prostatectomy without supplementary general anaesthesia.

Diagnostic

Intrathecal diamorphine has been used to determine whether chronic pain is genuine or whether there is a significant emotional element. As the onset of action of diamorphine is rapid, and the patient is unaware of the drug being injected, the test is also useful to determine whether patients are suitable for long-term treatment with intrathecal drugs (see page 91).

Obstetric

Intrathecal

Intrathecal diamorphine has been used for the relief of pain during labour (author's personal series). Although some of the patients had pain-free labour, others complained during delivery of the foetal head, and supplementary nitrous oxide and oxygen was necessary. In contrast to that seen with epidural bupivacaine, the pain of the contractions was diminished without loss of awareness of the contractions. There was no maternal cardiovascular or respiratory depression. The main disadvantage of intrathecal diamorphine was the short duration of action, 4–6 hours.

Epidural

Epidural bupivacaine is the commonest drug used to provide pain relief in labour. If the nerve block is incomplete, it can be rendered more effective by the addition of epidural fentanyl (Seebacher *et al.*, 1984). Following caesarian section under epidural bupivacaine, diamorphine 2–4 mg in 10 ml saline has been found to provide satisfactory postoperative relief for 24 hours.

Chronic pain and pain associated with terminal cancer

In patients with terminal cancer the aim is to have a patient who is alert, but with continuous pain suppression and with the fear and memory of pain abolished. Doses of drugs should be adequate and given before the effects of a previous injection have worn off, but, at the same time, an attempt should be made to increase the interval between the injections (Tuttle, 1985). Epidural and spinal routes of administration of opioids appear to be able to fulfil some of these aims and although morphine has been the most commonly-used drug, there is no valid reason why diamorphine should not produce satisfactory results, apart from its limited duration of action. If given by an infusion pump, the shorter duration would, in fact, be beneficial.

Arner and Arner (1985) administered epidural morphine in a daily dose of 4–480 mg by epidural catheter, tunnelled subcutaneously from the back to the anterior abdominal wall. Injections were made through a bacterial filter. Patients with deep-seated pain from carcinoma obtained relief, but those with cutaneous pain were unaffected. Another technique has involved connecting a spinal or epidural catheter to an Ommaya reservoir/pump, placed subcutaneously, which can be refilled with periodic injections of drugs.

Coombs *et al.*, 1983, have reported on the use of epidural and spinal morphine when the catheter was connected to an implanted infusion pump controlling the rate of administration of morphine. After the patients had been evaluated in hospital, to assess the amount of morphine required, the pump was programmed accordingly and each patient was allowed home, although a member of the family was trained to be aware of possible complications. The advantage of such reservoirs was that, even if their use did not produce complete freedom of pain, patients were able to reduce their oral requirements of analgesics. Wang, 1985, reported a 70% success rate in providing long-term pain relief with morphine, either by repeated injections or by an implanted pump. There was occasional mechanical failure of the pump, and sometimes tolerance to morphine developed. Respiratory depression was not a problem but somnolence, itching and sphincter disturbances were common.

Complications

Nausea and vomiting

Following intrathecal diamorphine there is a high incidence of nausea and vomiting in the first 24 hours, but there may be other causes for this, such as intravenous antibiotics. Also it may possibly be due to the direct action of the opioid on the vomiting centres in the floor of the fourth ventricle (see Fig. 6.5). In some patients (about 2%), nausea and vomiting persists for more than 24 hours.

Headache

Post-lumbar puncture headache is due to leakage of CSF into the epidural space with the consequent reduction in CSF pressure. It therefore depends on the size of the needle used. With 22–25 gauge needles (personal series), we found the incidence of headache to be less than 3% (see Fig. 6.5).

Pruritus

Itching is noted in patients after epidural or spinal opioids (Fig. 6.5). It may

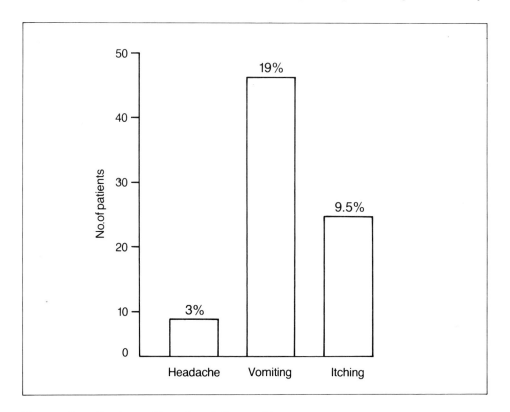

Fig. 6.5 Complications of intrathecal diamorphine.

be segmentally distributed, but is often generalised and affects a particular facial area (usually the nose). Although it does not appear to be caused by histamine release, it may respond to antihistamine drugs such as chlorpheniramine. However the most effective treatment is intramuscular or intravenous naloxone (0.1–0.2 mg).

Urinary retention

There have been numerous reports of urinary retention following epidural opioids and it appears that they may cause a decrease in detrusor pressure while increasing sphincteric tone in the bladder (Husted *et al.*, 1985). Urinary retention readily responds to naloxone.

Neurological sequelae

There have been no reported cases of neurological damage that can be ascribed directly to epidural or intraspinal diamorphine. This is in contrast to the incidence of neurological sequelae following spinal or extradural analgesia with local anaesthetics, though these drugs have been in use for much longer. Mehnert *et al.*, 1983, have reported a case of flaccid paralysis following epidural opioids in a patient who was also receiving heparin.

Respiratory depression

This is the most serious complication of intraspinal opioids. There have been many reports of respiratory depression with epidural or intrathecal morphine occurring approximately 4–17 hours after administration. The timing of this depression may be due to the slow absorption of morphine, but is more likely to be due to the cranial spread of the drug in the CSF, an action which is enhanced by its relatively poor lipid solubility. Diamorphine, having a much higher lipid solubility, is theoretically less liable to exhibit this delayed respiratory depression.

There is also the possibility that the profound peripheral effects in the dorsal horn reduce afferent stimulation and therefore respiratory drive is depressed. Bromage *et al.*, 1982, suggested that extradural morphine reached the brain stem and fourth ventricle 6 hours after administration, either by direct spread after diffusing into the CSF, or by absorption via the epidural veins. Positioning of the patient in the head-up posture appears to offer little protection against respiratory depression. Studies on CSF levels of opioids given spinally confirm the view that the drugs have a central action (Gourlay *et al.*, 1985; Max *et al.*, 1985).

It may well be, as suggested above, that diamorphine is a much safer drug in that, being lipophilic, it has a rapid onset and shorter duration, with less possibility of cranial spread. The insidious action of morphine on respiration presents serious problems in monitoring patients' respiration.

Intramuscular injections of morphine produce a peak concentration in the CSF 3 hours after injection, but after epidural administration the concentrations are 100 times greater (Nordberg *et al.*, 1985).

Thus care is necessary in the management of patients who have had intrathecal or epidural opioids, and it is suggested that all patients who have had major surgery should be monitored closely for at least 24 hours. Non-invasive methods include the use of inductance or impedance plethysmography. The introduction of pulse oximeters has made the detection of hypoxaemia easier to detect.

Postoperative respiratory depression can be prevented by meticulous attention to technique. If intrathecal diamorphine is used to provide intraoperative and postoperative pain relief, then supplementary intravenous analgesics should be avoided at operation, and the first intramuscular dose of analgesia given in the postoperative period should be in reduced dose, with care being taken to monitor respiration. Respiratory depression may be treated with intravenous naloxone 0.2–0.4 mg. As the duration of naloxone is short, subsequent doses may be required either intravenously or intramuscularly. However, naloxone, while reversing respiratory depression, does not affect the analgesia produced by spinal opioids (Jones and Jones, 1980). Nalbuphine has also been reported to increase respiratory activity following use of extradural diamorphine (Hammond, 1984).

Conclusion

Diamorphine has many attributes which render it a comparatively safe drug to be used for intraspinal techniques. Not only does intrathecal diamorphine provide intraoperative and postoperative analgesia it also suppresses the endocrine response to surgery. It may be used in the diagnosis of pain in obstetrics as well as alleviating chronic pain and the pain associated with terminal cancer. There are complications associated with intrathecal opioids, but these appear to be less with diamorphine when compared with other drugs.

References

Acalouschi, I., Ene, V., Lorinczi, E. and Nicolaus, F., (1986), 'Saddle block with pethidine for perineal operations', *British Journal of Anaesthesia*, **58**, 1,012.

Arner, S. and Arner, B., (1985), 'Differential effects of epidural morphine in the treatment of cancer-related pain', *Acta Anaesthesiologica Scandinavica*, **29**, 23.

Bailey, P. M., and Sangwan, S., (1986), 'Caudal analgesia for peri-anal surgery', *Anaesthesia*, **41**, 499.

Barron, D. and Strong, J. E., (1984), 'The safety and efficacy of intrathecal diamorphine', *Pain*, **18**, 279.

Bromage, P. R., Camporesi, E. M., Durant, P. A. C. and Neilson, C. H., (1982), 'Rostral spread of epidural morphine', *Anesthesiology*, **565**, 431.

Child, C. and Kaufman, L., (1985), 'Effect of intrathecal diamorphine on the adrenocortical, hyperglycaemic and cardiovascular responses to major colonic surgery', *British Journal of Anaesthesia*, **57**, 389.

Coombs, D. W., Saunders, R. L., Gaylor, M. and Pageau, M. G., (1982), 'Epidural narcotic infusion reservoir: implantation technique and efficacy', *Anesthesiology*, **59**, 469–73.

Coombs, D. W., Saunders, R. L., Gaylor, M. S., Block, A. R., Colton, T., Harbaugh, R., Pageau, M. G. and Mroz, W., (1983), 'Relief of continuous chronic pain by intraspinal narcotics infusion via an implanted reservoir', *Journal of the American Medical Association*, **250**, 2,336.

Cousins, M. J. and Mather, L. E., (1984), 'Intrathecal and epidural administration of opioids', *Anesthesiology*, **61**, 276.

Cozian, A., Pinaud, M., Lepage, J. Y., Lhoste, F. and Souron, R., (1986), 'Effects of meperidine spinal anesthesia on hemodynamics, plasma catecholamines, angiotensin I, aldosterone and histamine concentrations in elderly men', *Anesthesiology*, **64**, 815.

Feldberg, W., (1959), 'A physiological approach to the problem of general anaesthesia and loss of consciousness', *British Medical Journal*, **2**, 771.

Gourlay, G. K., Cherry, D. A. and Cousins, M. J., (1985), 'Cephalad migration of morphine in CSF following lumbar epidural administration in patients with cancer pain', *Pain*, **23**, 317.

Hammond, J. E., (1984), 'Reversal of opioid-associated late-onset respiratory depression by nalbuphine hydrochloride', *Lancet*, **ii**, 1,208.

Hjortsø, N. C., Lund, C., Mogensen, R., Bigler, D. and Kehlet, H., (1986), 'Epidural morphine improves pain relief and maintains sensory analgesia during continuous epidural bupivacaine after abdominal surgery', *Anesthesia and Analgesia*, **65**, 1,033.

Husted, S., Djurhuus, J. C., Husegaard, H. C. and Mortensen, J., (1985), 'Effect of postoperative extradural morphine on lower urinary tract function', *Acta Anaesthesiologica Scandinavica*, **29**, 183.

Jacobson, L., Phillips, P. D., Hull, C. J. and Conacher, I. D., (1983), 'On-demand analgesia. A double-blind comparison of on-demand intravenous fentanyl with regular intramuscular morphine', *Anaesthesia*, **38**, 10.

Jones, R. D. M. and Jones, J. G., (1980), 'Intrathecal morphine: naloxone reverses respiratory depression but not analgesia', *British Medical Journal*, **281**, 645.

Kaufman, L. and Bailey, P. M., (1987), 'Intravenous bumetanide attenuates the rise in plasma vasopressin concentrations during major surgical operations', *British Journal of Clinical Pharmacology*, **23**, 237.

Kaufman, L., (1981), 'Intrathecal heroin', *Lancet*, **ii**, 1,341.

Kotob, H. I. M., Hand, C. W., Moore, R. A., Evans, P. J. D., Wells, J., Rubin, A. P. and McQuay, H. J., (1986), 'Intrathecal morphine and heroin in humans. Six hour drug levels in spinal fluid and plasma', *Anesthesia and Analgesia*, **65**, 718.

Martin, W. R., Eades, C. G., Thompson, J. A., Huppler, R. E. and Gilbert, P. E., (1976), 'The effect of morphine and nalorphine-like drugs in the non-dependent and morphine-dependent chronic spinal dog', *Journal of Pharmacology and Experimental Therapeutics*, **197**, 517.

Martin, W. R., (1984), 'Pharmacology of opioids', *Pharmacological Review*, **35**, 285.

Max, M. B., Inturrisi, C. E., Kaiko, R. F., Grabinski, P. Y., Li, C. H. and Foley, K. M., (1985), 'Epidural and intrathecal opiates: cerebrospinal fluid and plasma profiles in patients with chronic cancer pain', *Clinical Pharmacology and Therapeutics*, **38**, 631.

Mehnert, J. H., Dupont, T. J. and Rose, D. H., (1983), 'Intermittent epidural morphine instillation for control of postoperative pain', *The American Journal of Surgery*, **146**, 145.

Moore, A., Bullingham, R., McQuay, H., Allen, M., Baldwin, D. and Cole, A., (1984), 'Spinal fluid kinetics of morphine and heroin', *Clinical Pharmacology and Therapeutics*, **35**, 40.

Nordberg, G., Borg, L., Hedner, R. and Mellstrand, T., (1985), 'CSF and plasma pharmacokinetics of intramuscular morphine', *European Journal of Clinical Pharmacology*, **27**, 677.

Phillips, D. M., Moore, R. A., Bullingham, R. E. S., Allen, M. C., Baldwin, D., Fisher, A., Lloyd, J. W. and McQuay, H. J., (1984), 'Plasma morphine concentrations and clinical effects after thoracic extradural morphine or diamorphine', *British Journal of Anaesthesia*, **56**, 829.

Seebacher, J., Henry, M., Galli-Douani, and Viars, P., (1984), 'Epidural opioids in labour. Regional Anaesthesia 1884–1984', Scott, D. B., McClure, J. and Wildsmith, J. A. W. (eds), (Sodertalje, Sweden, Information Consulting Medical, p. 111).

Staren, E. D. and Cullen, M. L., (1986), 'Epidural catheter analgesia for the management of post-operative pain', *Surgery, Gynaecology and Obstetrics*, **162**, 389.

Tuttle, C. B., (1985), 'Drug management of pain in cancer patients', *Canadian Medical Association Journal*, **132**, 121.

Wang, J. K., (1985), 'Intrathecal morphine for intractable pain secondary to cancer of pelvic organs', *Pain*, **21**, 99.

Wang, J. K., Nauss, L. E. and Thomas, J. E., (1979), 'Pain relief by intrathecally applied morphine in man', *Anesthesiology*, **50**, 149.

Watson, J., Moore, A., McQuay, H., Teddy, P., Baldwin, D., Allen, M. and Bullingham, R., (1984), 'Plasma morphine concentrations and analgesic effects of lumbar extradural morphine and heroin', *Anesthesia and Analgesia*, **63**, 629.

Williams, A. R., (1984), 'The pharmacist's approach to spinal analgesia', *Anaesthesia Review*, **2**, Kaufman, L. (ed), (London, Churchill Livingstone, p. 148).

Yaksh, T. L., (1981), 'Spinal opiate analgesia: characteristics and principles of action', *Pain*, **11**, 293.

Yaksh, T. L. and Rudy, T. A., (1976), 'Analgesia mediated by direct spinal action of narcotics', *Science*, **192**, 1,357.

ALEX T. PROUDFOOT, BSc, FRCPE

7 Diamorphine overdosage

Circumstances of overdosage

Diamorphine overdosage may arise in three different ways.

Abuse for pleasure

Abuse for pleasurable or recreational purposes is probably the commonest cause of acute diamorphine overdosage in present-day society. In this situation, the drug is most likely to be administered intravenously ('mainlined') although, in some areas at least, a return to smoking and inhalation is becoming increasingly fashionable. The latter at least makes the possibility of massive acute overdose remote. In contrast, accidental overdosage is an ever-present risk of mainlining and is probably due to inexperience or to unexpected increases in the potency of street drug. The latter arises when increased availability of high-quality drug reduces the need for suppliers to 'cut' (dilute) what is sold on the streets to the same extent. In the preceding lean period, users may have learned to increase the amounts they inject so that they can continue to experience a 'rush' and obviously there is a serious risk of accidental overdosage if the same quantity is used but the potency is greater. One study in Atlanta, USA, showed that peaks of heroin deaths correlated with the potency of street drug (Alexander, 1974).

Misadventure while 'body packing'

The term 'body packing' refers to smuggling drugs by making them into parcels small enough to be swallowed for later retrieval from vomitus or faeces or for insertion into the rectum or vagina ('stuffing'). While the size of packets can obviously vary considerably, a surprisingly large number can be concealed in this way. Up to 103, each the size of a small egg, and with a combined weight of over 580 g, were reported in one fatal case (Joynt and Mikhael, 1985). The courier is clearly at risk of massive acute overdosage should one or more packets rupture or if the nature of the wrapping allows the contents to leach out (Arora *et al.*, 1982). The latter is clearly critical. A number of materials, including cellophane and foil, have been used but condoms appear to be the most popular. Only the highest quality and, correspondingly, potentially the most toxic drugs are likely to be transported in this way. The purity of the diamorphine in some Australian cases varied from 29–85% (Dunne, 1983). One presumes that the financial rewards compensate for the considerable hazards of this technique.

Therapeutic overdosage

Therapeutic overdosage is most likely to occur in elderly people who have severe pain, as from myocardial infarction or a similarly distressing acute illness, and particularly if they are frail. In such cases, the usual initial intravenous dose of 5 mg may be excessive, and half that dose may be sufficient (*British National Formulary*, 1987).

Features of overdosage

Three features are the hallmarks of overdosage with diamorphine, as with the other opioid analgesics: impairment of consciousness, respiratory depression and miosis. Indeed, no other drug or group of drugs produces this diagnostic triad of signs. The depth of coma is obviously variable but it usually correlates with the degree of respiratory depression. The latter may be manifest by reduced depth of breathing (low tidal volume), but more characteristically bradypnoea is the striking abnormality. Respiratory rates of 4–6/minute are not uncommon in severe overdosage and presage apnoea. While the depth of coma and extent of reduction of the respiratory rate reflect the severity of poisoning, the size of the pupils does not; even therapeutic doses of diamorphine cause them to become pin-point, probably because of stimulation of the parasympathetic nerve supply to the iris.

Severe overdosage

Severe diamorphine overdosage is frequently fatal, and most deaths occur outside hospital and without the victim having received any form of medical care. A minority reach hospital within minutes of cardio-respiratory arrest but most will be breathing spontaneously. They will usually be deeply unconscious, unresponsive to painful stimuli, and have an absent cough reflex with generalised hypotonia and hyporeflexia. The respiratory rate will be markedly reduced and deep cyanosis and hypotension are common. Arterial blood gas analysis at this stage can be expected to show a low pO_2 and a raised pCO_2, the combination of the two leading to a mixed metabolic/respiratory acidosis. As noted above, the pupils will be pin-point unless hypoxia has become dominant and they begin to dilate.

Suspicion of diamorphine overdosage should prompt examination of the antecubital fossae, feet and groins for injection sites. Signs of pulmonary oedema may be present in the most severe cases (see page 100) and, rarely, convulsions may occur.

Mild to moderate overdosage

Since most diamorphine overdosage is the result of illicit use and intoxication is the objective, mild to moderate poisoning is unlikely to come to medical notice. Even individuals who become unconscious may not be referred for medical help but simply observed or given rudimentary 'care' by their less intoxicated fellow users until consciousness is regained or it becomes clear that something serious is amiss. Not uncommonly there may be delays of several hours during which hypotension and hypoxia can cause irreversible brain damage.

Mostly mildly intoxicated patients will be conscious and communicative, if somewhat drowsy, euphoric and slow to respond. Respiration is unlikely to be impaired but miosis will be present and there may be nystagmus on lateral gaze.

Interactions with other drugs

The toxicity of diamorphine in overdosage will be potentiated by virtually any other central nervous system depressant drug, including alcohol and the benzodiazepines, which are so widely used in present-day society. Addicts in particular are likely to use two or more psychotropic drugs simultaneously, and it has been clearly shown that the risk of death from diamorphine abuse is significantly greater in those who consume alcohol at the same time (Ruttenber and Luke, 1984; Morbidity and Mortality Weekly Report, 1983) although it is acknowledged that other factors may also be important.

Complications

Diamorphine overdosage carries a number of complications, the incidence of which has not been defined.

Pulmonary oedema

Pulmonary oedema is probably the most important complication of diamorphine overdosage and is present in more than half of fatal cases. It is also well-documented in severe, non-fatal overdosage, but is probably uncommon. Its aetiology is poorly understood but the oedema is thought to be of the increased pulmonary capillary permeability type rather than due to cardiac causes, since pulmonary arterial wedge pressures are normal. Almost certainly it is similar to the non-cardiac pulmonary oedema seen in other forms of acute poisoning, notably with salicylates.

In its most florid form, there will be obvious respiratory distress with deep cyanosis, and foam may pour from the nostrils and mouth. Crepitations may or may not be present throughout both lungs and the patient will show all the other features of severe poisoning. The diagnosis is usually obvious from the chest radiograph. At the other extreme, some patients with diamorphine-induced pulmonary oedema may be conscious and asymptomatic (Steinberg and Karliner, 1968).

Rhabdomyolysis

Necrosis of skeletal muscle, particularly in the limbs, is a well-documented complication of diamorphine overdosage (Nicholls *et al.*, 1982; Trewby *et al.*, 1981). Its aetiology is almost certainly multifactorial. Prolonged immobility while comatose, particularly if it occurs within confined spaces, with the arms and legs being compressed by external objects, and by the victim's other limbs, trunk and head, is probably the most important factor. However, convulsions, hypotension, acidosis, hypoxia and possibly a direct-drug effect, may all have a role.

Hyperpyrexia, hyperkalaemia, hyperphosphataemia, hypocalcaemia and hyperuricaemia are common metabolic abnormalities in the initial phases. Plasma creatine kinase activity is grossly elevated and myoglobinuria will be present in some cases, making the urine brown or 'claret' coloured, according to pH. Acute renal failure due to tubular necrosis may follow in turn.

The diagnosis of rhabdomyolysis requires a high index of suspicion. Signs of damage may not be obvious at the stage when decompression of muscle compartments might be helpful. Once the patient recovers consciousness, however, pain is a most compelling symptom, and the affected limb may have become oedematous, tight and bruised.

Complications resulting from the method of abuse

A considerable number of complications of diamorphine overdosage have been reported which are due more probably to the consequences of the method of abuse rather than to the drug itself. They include viral and bacterial infections such as hepatitis B, human immuno-deficiency virus infection, bacterial endocarditis, thrombophlebitis, abscesses and systemic candidiasis; emboli to the retina, lungs and digits; and major central nervous system damage such as spongiform leucoencephalopathy and a variety of spinal cord lesions. These will not be discussed further.

Complications due to contaminants in the diamorphine

Some of the apparent complications of diamorphine overdosage may also be due to the numerous substances which are used to 'cut' (dilute) drug before it is sold on the street. Almost certainly some of these, such as talc, contribute to the long-term, progressive, granulomatous embolic lesions while others, particularly quinine, may be responsible for some of the more acute toxic phenomena.

Management

General

Clinicians must regretfully conclude that, unless the patient is elderly and clearly poisoned as a result of therapeutic overdosage, every patient must be regarded as a heroin abuser and therefore a possible hazard to others by virtue of being a carrier of hepatitis B or human immuno-deficiency viruses. As a minimum, those handling the patient should wear gloves, particularly if major medical intervention is required and there is likely to be contact with blood, saliva, urine and faeces. Special care must be taken to avoid stabbing oneself with needles contaminated with the patient's blood, and these and excreta should be disposed of appropriately. Apart from this warning, the medical management of the patient poisoned with heroin is relatively easy. It has been transformed by the advent of opioid antagonists, although these are not essential to complete recovery. Supportive care alone could suffice, but recovery would take considerably longer.

Cardiopulmonary resuscitation

Patients who are in cardiorespiratory arrest when first seen should be resuscitated using the well-established techniques. Measures specific to heroin are not essential at this stage, but naloxone should be given as soon as practicable since it may abort the need for prolonged periods of intensive care.

Naloxone

Naloxone is a pure opioid antagonist and is the treatment of choice for heroin overdosage.

Dosage and routes of administration

Naloxone is usually given intravenously or intramuscularly, the former route being preferable in crisis situations. The dose for an adult is a minimum of 0.8 mg and preferably 1.2 mg, while that for a child is 10 μg/kg body weight. Alternatively, it may be administered by the endotracheal route (Tandberg, 1982), or injected sub-lingually (Rappolt et al., 1980) if venous access is impossible and the clinical situation desperate. Larger doses may occasionally be required.

Naloxone has the disadvantage that its plasma half-life is short (30–60 minutes) and repeated doses may be required to prevent addicts from lapsing back into coma and respiratory depression after initial treatment. Intravenous infusion of naloxone at a rate sufficient to keep the patient conscious has therefore been recommended, but while this may be a useful adjunct to management, it is not a substitute for regular and frequent clinical review and administration of extra bolus doses as indicated. Addicts whose heroin overdosage is completely reversed by the initial dose of naloxone and who insist on leaving the emergency department immediately are at particular risk of recurrence of opioid toxicity, and are best given an additional intramuscular dose of naloxone before leaving.

Clinical effects

Doses such as those recommended above can confidently be expected to reverse diamorphine toxicity completely in little more than a minute. Failure to respond is evidence of the involvement of another central nervous system depressant drug, or the presence of brain damage. Following reversal, the respiratory rate frequently rises above normal for a period with consequent hyperventilation, as was clearly illustrated by one of the early papers on its use (Evans et al., 1973). The reasons for the overshoot phenomenon are not clear, but it may be the result of unmasking physical dependence.

Adverse effects

The side effects of naloxone are few. The only consistent hazards in the context of heroin overdosage are that the symptom(s) for which it was given in the first place may return unabated and, in addicts, an acute withdrawal state may be precipitated. However, the short half-life of naloxone ensures that the withdrawal state is correspondingly brief, usually less than two hours. Indeed, it has been so valuable, and relatively free from adverse effects, that its 'blind' use in undiagnosed coma has been widely advocated, assuming other readily-reversible causes such as hypoglycaemia have been excluded. Inevitably, such indiscriminate use has attracted critics who point to the occasional reports of ventricular fibrillation (Cuss *et al.*, 1984) and pulmonary oedema (Prough *et al.*, 1984) complicating justified use. On the evidence available, the advantages of relatively free use of naloxone appear to outweigh the very infrequent serious adverse effects.

Specificity of the response to naloxone

The specificity of the response to naloxone is in some doubt. In patients where there is uncertainty about heroin being responsible for coma, naloxone or another antagonist should be given and its effect on the cardinal signs of toxicity assessed. If narcotic analgesics are the cause, the improvement in the level of consciousness may be dramatic, and patients have been known to awake from deep coma and remove the endotracheal tubes inserted earlier during resuscitation. Equally promptly, the pupils dilate and the respiratory rate increases. These effects are usually apparent within 1–2 minutes. Early experience suggested that naloxone did not change the level of consciousness, respiratory rate, minute volume or pupil size when used in non-narcotic poisoning (Evans *et al.*, 1973), but, since then, there have been a number of reports indicating that it may partially reverse toxicity due to ethanol, benzodiazepines and other drugs (Handal *et al.*, 1983). Even a non-specific arousal action has been postulated. However, these responses are unpredictable and a dramatic improvement is strong evidence in favour of opioid overdosage.

Other antagonists

Naloxone has superseded the older narcotic antagonists but, unfortunately, not all countries can afford to use it. Nalorphine hydrochloride is still used in some third world countries and is extremely effective in definite diamorphine overdosage. It can be given intravenously or intramuscularly in doses of 5–10 mg, repeated if necessary. However, nalorphine has partial agonist actions in addition to antagonist effects, and must be given with care because excessive amounts may depress the central nervous system and respiration. Even therapeutic amounts of nalorphine may potentiate the effects of non-narcotic psychotropic drugs, and it should not be used in overdosage with them. Similarly, its use as a diagnostic test is not without risk.

Naltrexone is one of the most recent additions to the range of opioid antagonists but is not yet available in the UK. Naltrexone has minimal agonist actions and can be given orally as well as parenterally, making it suitable for long-term management of addiction (Ginzburg and Mac-Donald, 1987). Its role in the treatment of acute diamorphine overdosage has yet to be defined, although its oral effectiveness, and a plasma half-life of about eight hours, makes it a potentially attractive adjunct to the treatment of the addict who insists on leaving the emergency department immediately the effects of diamorphine have been reversed by naloxone.

Supportive care

Administration of opioid antagonists is not essential for recovery from diamorphine overdosage, although there is no argument that the process would take considerably longer and require a much greater level of intensive care than would be necessary if drugs were used. The supportive measures which are required are as follows.

Airway and ventilation

A clear airway must be established as a matter of urgency. Secretions and vomitus should be removed from the mouth by whatever means are at hand, and a short oro-pharyngeal airway inserted, if one is available. The patient should then be turned into the semi-prone position. If the cough reflex is abolished and the appropriate expertise and equipment are available, a cuffed endotracheal tube should be inserted. The chest should then be carefully auscultated to ensure good air entry into both lungs, in case the tube has gone too far down and into the right main bronchus, or has been inserted into the oesophagus. Adequate warming and humidification of the inspired air is essential in patients who are intubated.

Peripheral circulatory failure

In many cases clearing the airway and improving ventilation will be all the action that is required to produce an increase in blood pressure and tissue perfusion. However, if hypotension persists despite these measures, the first step should be to elevate the feet 15 cm above the trunk to increase the venous return to the heart. Should this be ineffective, a central venous line should be inserted and the intravascular volume expanded with colloid as necessary. Only a very small minority will need inotropic agents, such as dopamine and dobutamine, in addition to these measures.

Pulmonary oedema

Patients with diamorphine-induced pulmonary oedema can often be managed conservatively, provided it is not too severe, and blood gas tensions can be monitored as frequently as is indicated by changes in the patient's clinical state. Oxygen should be given in concentrations sufficient to maintain a normal arterial oxygen tension, or at least one which will ensure the greatest possible haemoglobin oxygen saturation. In the most severe cases, spontaneous respiration is unlikely to achieve acceptable arterial blood gas tensions, and endotracheal intubation and assisted ventilation with positive end-expiratory pressure, will be required until the oedema clears.

Body packing

The vagina can be cleared of packets relatively easily and safely but attempts at manual evacuation of the rectum may lead to rupture of packets and systemic toxicity from rectal absorption. In these cases, laxatives are probably all that are indicated and most packets can be expected to pass spontaneously. Packets which have been ingested but remain within the stomach may be retrieved by inducing emesis (Robins and Ray, 1986), but the management of those which have passed through the pylorus is controversial. The current trend is towards as conservative an approach as possible, surgery only being indicated if obstructive features develop, or if intra-abdominal packets rupture and cause systemic toxicity. The majority of cases should simply be observed while given laxatives or other measures to encourage transit through the gut (Caruana *et al.*, 1984; McCarron and Wood, 1983).

Conclusion

Diamorphine overdosage occasionally is due to therapeutic misadventure but is more commonly due to misuse of diamorphine diluted with a variety of inert substances. Impairment of consciousness, bradypnoea and miosis are the diagnostic hallmarks of overdosage and can be reversed almost immediately by adequate doses of naloxone. Rhabdomyolysis may complicate severe poisoning and non-cardiogenic pulmonary oedema is frequently found in fatal cases. The present trend towards smoking heroin rather than injecting it may reduce the morbidity and mortality from overdosage.

References

Alexander, M., (1974), 'Surveillance of heroin-related deaths in Atlanta, 1971 to 1973', *Journal of the American Medical Association*, **229**, 677.

Arora, S., Tafreshi, M., Sobo, S., Krochmal, P. and Alexander, L. L., (1982), 'Accidental overdose intoxication: a hazard of drug smuggling', *Journal of National Medical Association*, **74**, 663.

British National Formulary, (1987), **13**, 171.

Caruana, D. S., Weinback, B., Goerg, D. and Gardner, L. B., (1984), 'Cocaine packet ingestion', *Annals of Internal Medicine*, **100**, 73.

Cuss, F. M., Colaco, C. J. and Baron, J. H., (1984), 'Cardiac arrest after reversal of effects of opiates with naloxone', *British Medical Journal*, **288**, 363.

Dunne, J. W., (1983), 'Drug smuggling by internal body concealment', *Medical Journal of Australia*, **2**, 436.

Evans, L. E. J., Roscoe, P., Swainson, C. P. and Prescott, L. F., (1973), 'Treatment of drug overdosage with naloxone, a specific narcotic antagonist', *Lancet*, **i**, 452.

Ginzburg, H. M. and MacDonald, M. G., (1987), 'The role of naloxone in the management of drug abuse', *Medical Toxicology*, **2**, 83.

Handal, K. A., Schauben, J. L. and Salamone, F. R., (1983), 'Naloxone', *Annals of Emergency Medicine*, **12**, 438.

Joynt, B. P. and Mikhael, N. Z., (1985), 'Sudden death of a heroin body packer', *Journal of Analytical Toxicology*, **9**, 238.

McCarron, M. M. and Wood, J. D., (1983), 'The cocaine "body packer" syndrome', *Journal of the American Medical Association*, **350**, 1,417.

1983 Morbidity and Mortality Weekly Report, Centers for Disease Control, 'Heroin-related deaths – District of Columbia, 1980–1982', *Journal of the American Medical Association*, **250**, 463.

Nicholls, K., Niall, J. F. and Moran, J. E., (1982), 'Rhabdomyolysis and renal failure: complications of narcotic abuse, *Medical Journal of Australia*, **2**, 387.

Prough, D. S., Roy, R., Bumgarner, J. and Shannon, G., (1984), 'Acute pulmonary edema in healthy teenagers following conservative doses of intravenous naloxone', *Anesthesiology*, **60**, 485.

Rappolt, R. T., Gay, G. R., Decker, W. J. and Inaba, D. S., (1980), 'NAGD regimen for the coma of drug-related overdose', *Annals of Emergency Medicine*, **9**, 357.

Robins, J. B. and Rae, P. W., (1986), 'Recovery of ingested heroin packets', *Archives of Emergency Medicine*, **3**, 125.

Ruttenber, A. J. and Luke, J. L., (1984), 'Heroin-related deaths: new epidemiological insights', *Science*, **226**, 14.

Steinberg, A. D. and Karliner, J. S., (1968), 'The clinical spectrum of heroin pulmonary oedema', *Archives of Internal Medicine*, **122**, 122.

Tandberg, D., (1982), 'Treatment of heroin overdose with endotracheal naloxone', *Annals of Emergency Medicine*, **11**, 443.

Trewby, P. N., Kalfayan, P. Y. and Elkeles, R. S., (1981), 'Heroin and hyperkalaemia', *Lancet*, **i**, 327.

J. ROY ROBERTSON, MRCGP

8 Diamorphine abuse and addiction

Current situation in the United Kingdom

The global picture of diamorphine abuse since World War II has shown a pattern of epidemics, occurring in different places at different times, followed by endemic patterns of use made up of individuals who started to use the drug during the epidemic phase, followed by a comparatively small number of new recruits. This is followed some time later by further epidemics, often in separate localities. Thus, in Europe in general, and in the United Kingdom in particular, we are witnessing a number of centres of diamorphine abuse, from which a spread to outlying districts occurs. The United States of America, however, which has a large endemic problem of diamorphine use, has not seen these new epidemic patterns of the 1980s. If those using diamorphine in the UK in the present decade are to follow a pattern similar to their American counterparts, then the situation in Britain in ten years' time may be similar to that in the USA now.

Estimates are notoriously unreliable in terms of the numbers misusing the drug at any one time. The Home Office figures (1984) in Britain recorded 7,400 diamorphine users – a steady rise since the beginning of the decade. Official sources, however, estimate a multiplication factor of 5–10 to arrive at a more realistic number in the UK (DHSS, 1982), and Government sources (House of Commons report, 1985) variously quote figures of 40–100,000 individuals using diamorphine on an intermittent or continuing basis. These individuals are reported to be younger and to have a higher percentage of females than in previous UK and current US studies (Stimson and Oppenheimer, 1982; Vaillant, 1973).

In the UK there are many regional variations in regard to the types of drugs abused, and the methods of administration, for instance, by injection or by smoking. This has given rise to certain apparently unique situations where local problems have emerged that have not been reported elsewhere. Examples of this are infections such as hepatitis B, acquired immunodeficiency syndrome (AIDS), eye infections, endocarditis and many others. Other drugs used in combination with diamorphine are equally variable, reflecting local legal and illegal practice. Overdoses occur in groups rather than evenly through time (Kaplan, 1983; Bucknall and Robertson, 1986) and may be associated with the availability and abuse of other drugs such as dipipanone (Diconal), buprenorphine (Temgesic), barbiturates, dextropropoxyphene and methadone, all of which, when taken in combination with diamorphine, can have an additional respiratory depressant effect.

Even before the emerging awareness of the human immunodeficiency virus (HIV) infection as a major risk to drug-takers, there were early indications that local epidemics in the UK were past their peak (Robertson and Bucknall, 1986). The rapid escalation in knowledge of AIDS exposure in drug-injectors will presumably have an impact on those using diamorphine. It will certainly account for many premature deaths in the near future, and will change the pattern of behaviour among diamorphine-users, possibly with a move to abstinence in some.

The singular importance of drug injectors in the AIDS pandemic is their potential for spreading the disease from the so-called 'high-risk groups' of homosexual men, blood product recipients, and drug users, into the general population. This risk occurs as the majority of known drug injectors are heterosexual and many are female, according to official reports (Home Office). Once this virus is present in these individuals, it may spread rapidly to non-drug using males and females, and children born to infected mothers.

Natural history of addiction

Established theory about the natural history of diamorphine addiction is based on the work of Winick, 1962, and Waldorf, 1972, and subsequent elaboration of the concepts of maturing out of drug use, and spontaneous remission resulting from environmental and domestic circumstances. Contrary to the common belief that diamorphine misuse leads almost inevitably to permanent addiction, long-term follow up studies have shown that fifty per cent or more of individuals have remained abstinent even after several years of misuse (Vaillant, 1973). Thorley, 1981, suggests that many may stop using diamorphine after only a short history of use.

Recent information that the present cohort of drug-users consists of heavy users, not-so-heavy users, and those who use the drug on a more or less experimental basis, has further challenged the permanence, continuation and inevitable outcome of heroin dependence (Zinberg, 1979, 1984). Stimson's, 1982, view that there are various categories of heroin users, based, presumably, on personality, circumstance and environment, has failed in the past to change the notion that all drug users are the same and therefore require the same therapy.

Nevertheless, this information and that reported by Robins, 1976, from the data emerging from the Vietnam Veterans' studies, leads to a modification of the 'once an addict always an addict' thesis, and indeed, only a minority seem to live up to this prediction.

Outcome, therefore, for any one individual is not easy to predict in the short term, and prognostic markers identifying those who might respond to any specific therapy, are so far elusive. Certainly, in the short term, reliable methods of achieving abstinence are absent. Studies observing the therapeutic options taken up by groups of drug users demonstrate that the majority of individuals avail themselves of several of these treatments in the course of their drug-using career. General practitioners, psychiatrists, physicians, family, friends, associates, voluntary group workers, residential agencies, social workers and many others are amongst those who attempt to exert influence on most diamorphine-users. While many claim some success, there is no evidence that any one approach can produce consistent results.

In follow-up studies of groups of individuals using diamorphine, somewhere between 1–2% die per annum of drug-related causes (Robertson and Bucknall, 1986; Thorley, 1981; Zinberg, 1979; Robins, Heker and Denis, 1976; and Joe, Lehman and Simpson, 1982). This represents a considerable mortality compared to non-drug using adults. Deaths are related most often to overdosage, infection, trauma and neglect, but AIDS may significantly overshadow all of these in the immediate future.

Dependence on diamorphine appears, therefore, to have a limited time span in many individuals. Those avoiding fatal consequences, more often by luck than design, may well achieve a more stable state after an initial damaging phase, and indeed may achieve permanent abstinence after a longer, or shorter, period of diamorphine use. The initial period may be the most damaging in terms of behaviour-related infections, and the survivors of this phase may well improve their life expectancy. The recovery period may involve many attempts at abstinence, or at comparatively controlled use. These episodes are described as 'practicing for abstinence' and represent a pathway to recovery which, if recognised, might be facilitated or encouraged by those in contact with the individual.

Diagnosis in general practice

Determining the onset of drug dependence in an individual is something which can only be done in retrospect, as he or she is clearly not dependent on diamorphine when taking the first inhalation or injection. Indeed it may be that many individuals indulge in the drug over long periods of time without ever achieving the status of dependence as defined in the 1971 Act (DHSS, 1984). For this reason, the terms 'addiction' and 'addict' are confusing, and confining oneself to the use of 'dependence' and 'drug-user' avoids this difficulty.

Diamorphine usage, being an illegal and therefore covert activity, may be undetected for months or years. Presentation to a general practitioner is most common when problems are encountered, or when relatives or friends become aware of behavioural change or difficulties. Thus presentation may be direct when an individual seeks advice or, more commonly, indirect when a symptom of diamorphine use reveals the underlying problem. Communication through a third party might often be the mode of presentation as, at least in the early stages, consequences of drug use are more obviously domestic and social rather than medical.

Nevertheless, the awareness of diamorphine use as a potential cause of all sorts of symptoms and signs is important to the physician. Behavioural, psychological, physical and domestic problems may become clear with this knowledge, and clinical signs and symptoms such as lassitude, weight loss, aches and pains, lymphadenopathy, jaundice, abdominal pains, tachycardia, heart murmurs and many others may have the same underlying cause. As in other disorders, the clinical suspicion and awareness of the possibility of drug abuse is the single most important factor in determining whether the diagnosis will be established early or late. The fact that most drug-users feel that it is to their advantage to declare their drug use may make the covert user less obvious but, at least in those injecting the drug, injection sites and toxicology testing will confirm the provisional diagnosis.

Those physicians working in areas of known high drug misuse will be aware of the casual patient registered at a temporary address, and requiring urgent analgesic for a painful condition, or the late-night call for obscure painful conditions in individuals displaying a remarkable insight into pharmaceutical products. The story that 'just doesn't sound right' or the pain that is atypical should arouse suspicion.

Presentation in general practice, therefore, may take many forms and serves to underline the variety of problems and individuals associated with illegal drug abuse. The response by the doctor must similarly be variable depending upon circumstance.

Complications

To enumerate the possible complications of diamorphine use is beyond the scope of this text. Suffice it to say that a multitude of disorders have been attributed to diamorphine use, usually from the acquisition of infection or toxic contaminants rather than the effects of the drug itself. Thus malaria, tetanus, brucellosis, septicaemia, endocarditis, hepatitis, AIDS, nephritis, brain abscess and toxoplasmosis have all been described and are mainly due to the ill-advised use of contaminated injecting equipment. Recently, epidemics of hepatitis B virus (with or without the delta agent) and HIV infection have been shown to spread rapidly through groups of drug injectors, and the evidence from Milan (Lazzarin *et al.*, 1985) and Edinburgh (Robertson *et al.*, 1986) of HIV spread, demonstrates just how rapid and complete this can be, given the right conditions.

The occurrence of endocarditis and ocular infection appears to be localised and determined by behaviour and local problems with a contaminated drug supply (Servant, 1984). The outbreak of endophthalmitis described in Glasgow was thought to be caused by proprietary lemon juice from plastic containers used to acidify diamorphine in the preparation of an intravenous shot. Left unrefrigerated the resultant culture of candida albicans allowed introduction of a bolus of infection.

Systemic infections, therefore, depend on local practices and conditions and are consequently variable in time and severity. They basically relate to ignorance or inability to observe adequate sterile conditions for injection.

Local complications at the injection site have a similar aetiology. In those with a regard for asepsis they can be surprisingly absent for many years. Damage to peripheral veins by blunt or infected needles can give rise to thrombosis and occlusion. Local sepsis may result in abscess formation, and irritant materials not designed for IV use can cause local damage which may or may not be infected.

Overdosage must represent the single most immediately damaging consequence of drug use, especially with intravenous drug abuse. The simplistic view that death by overdosage is caused by an excess of opioid in a non-tolerant user, or in one whose tolerance has been lost, does not account for some features of the problem. Well documented accounts of overdosage occurring after amounts of heroin that were previously safe, suggest that additional factors may be present. Tolerance to drugs may be variable, depending on environmental and psychological factors, and this adds another dimension to the understanding of the problem. Studies incriminating a second, third or fourth drug in the cause of death have highlighted the cumulative effect on the respiratory centre of such drugs as ethyl alcohol, dextropopoxyphene, buprenorphine, methadone and other opioids when present in the diamorphine user.

The preferential diagnosis of diamorphine abuse as the primary cause of death in a known user may obscure the presence of a second or third factor. Thus death from pneumonia, infection or poisoning by another drug may be recorded as death due to diamorphine, resulting in excessive notification as a cause of death with an under-notification of the underlying or associated cause.

Treatment and rehabilitation

In response to changing requirements brought about by increasing numbers of diamorphine users, and the presence of hepatitis B and AIDS viruses, the treatment of those taking illegal diamorphine has undergone many changes in recent years. This is a continuing trend and the influence of HIV infection will undoubtedly have a major effect. The presence of several approaches to treatment indicates that no single method has been proved to be superior, either in achieving abstinence or in being free from practical or theoretical complications. As with other behavioural disorders, the influence of changing attitudes in society must never be underestimated as a potent force in drug-taking, and in its management.

The treatment or management might best be divided into three areas, as follows, which may be used simultaneously or independently in any individual:
1. Treatment of the withdrawal syndrome.
2. Maintenance of dependence by substitution therapy.
3. Non-drug management and rehabilitation.

Treatment of the withdrawal syndrome

Drug withdrawal is the situation in which doctors find most contradictions and inconsistencies. Faced with a diamorphine-dependent individual with a desire, apparent or real, to achieve abstinence, the provision of adequate alternative drug substitution to achieve that condition seems logical. The doctor requires accurate information about the length and level of dependence (in money spent per day or grams of drug used) in order to make a decision on what to prescribe and for how long. The rapid and complete progression of the patient to the drug-free state may be a measure of the determination of the individual, the efficacy of the treatment, or a minimal degree of dependence. Conversely, prolonged and protracted withdrawal symptoms, or the more frequent relapse shortly after drug reduction or abstinence has been achieved, may be measures, equally, of lack of determination, the inadequacy of therapy, or a severe degree of dependence. It might also be a reflection of the insincerity of the approach by a patient during a period of non-availability of illicit drug, or a way of subsidising other income by reselling prescribed drugs. All these variables, and the frequency with which excuses for failure occur, lead the cautious practitioner to establish a set of rules or guidelines. The treatment of the withdrawal syndrome by any means at all should be associated with the recognition that relapse is likely, even in the most motivated patient, but that this does not necessarily represent failure.

Maintenance of dependence

This represents a different philosophy in the management of drug abuse and drug dependency. The acceptance in any individual that abstinence or control of drug-taking can only be achieved by alternative drug prescribing on a continuous basis, recognises many of the problems discussed above, but assumes that change is impossible. However, in some individuals, at some periods in their lives, maintenance of a stable state is best achieved by the legal supply of an opioid (e.g. oral methadone linctus BP). This allows for a period of assessment and treatment, with relief from criminal involvement and its associated domestic and financial stress.

Most countries which allow the legal provision of substitute drug insist that supervision shall be adequate, that there is no obvious abuse of the programme, that attempts are made to progress to abstinence in the long term, and that psychological and social supports are present to give help in moving in this direction.

Non-drug treatment and rehabilitation

The nature of the recent wave of diamorphine use in the UK has given rise to a requirement for local community services and agencies to advise and treat drug-abusers. Home Office statistics confirm the decreasing age and the increasing number of female diamorphine users. The predominance of reports from areas of high unemployment and low socio-economic performance, has required a change of direction by those agencies which provide support or therapy.

There is an increased awareness that withdrawal and rehabilitation can sometimes be managed by a non-prescribing regime. Many reports testify to the success of such regimes, based on social and psychological support rather than on the provision of alternative drugs. The advantage of this approach is that it eliminates those drug abusers who are less motivated or less able to cope with non-drug therapy. While this selection process means that these groups, or centres, are dealing with a different type of individual, it is also likely that they are dealing with drug users at a different stage in the natural development of the drug taking process.

It is essential to provide a range of services, drug related or non drug related, residential or non-residential, to fulfil the individual requirements at different stages in the life of any drug-abuser.

The somewhat confused information regarding regional variations in patterns of drug misuse, and the provision of therapeutic services, tends to give rise to variable approaches to the problem. Research based on psychiatric care is difficult to compare to that based on medical or social services, and such different perspectives are not always easy to combine to form an overall view of the problem.

Conclusion

The present situation is especially complicated because of its innovative stage. New requirements in the 1980s led to the evolution of a whole range of services and of professional workers. The old rigid views of what diamorphine-dependence was, and who those involved in the 1960s and 1970s were, has given way to a recognition that drug abusers often do not conform to any stereotype, and cannot be treated or managed in a uniform way. A different approach has been stimulated by the understanding that while remission and relapse are a common pattern of behaviour in most drug-takers, over a period of years the trend is nevertheless towards improvement (Robertson, 1987).

Finally, the presence of the HIV and hepatitis B virus has given a new intensity to these management problems. Paradoxically, the concern over AIDS may stimulate the trend towards a policy of risk reduction, rather than a demand for immediate abstinence from drug taking. This philosophy has undoubtedly been resisted by many in the medical and political establishments on the grounds that to suggest that diamorphine abuse is not a lethal habit is to encourage its use. However, it is because drug users continue to survive, despite all the potential dangers, that they have become a major mode of introduction of HIV into the non drug using heterosexual population. After a painful process of accepting the reality of diamorphine use in many provincial centres in the 1980s, the scene is now set for the provision of a range of services to cope with an ongoing problem.

The next ten years are likely to see a reduction in the numbers of new diamorphine users, and will identify the incidence of HIV and AIDS in this group. Some drug users, or potential users, who have refused to acknowledge the dangers of diamorphine itself, may now see that this new development poses a quite unacceptable risk. The effect of this disease on patterns of drug abuse remains speculative, but the requirement for an increased range of services for diamorphine users and their families remains a challenge not only for the health and social services, but for any agency or individual who is prepared to become involved.

References

Bucknall, A. B. V. and Robertson, J. R., (1986), 'Deaths of heroin users in a general practice population', *Journal of the Royal College of General Practitioners*, **36**, 120.

DHSS, (1982), 'Treatment and rehabilitation', *Report of the Advisory Council on the Misuse of Drugs*, (London, HMSO).

DHSS, (1984), 'Guidelines of good clinical practice in the treatment of drug misuse', *Report of the Medical Working Group on Drug Dependence*, (London, HMSO).

Home Office, (1984), 'Statistics of the misuse of drugs in the United Kingdom', *Home Office Statistical Bulletin*, (London, HMSO).

House of Commons, (Session 1984–1985), 'Misuse of drugs: with special reference to the treatment and rehabilitation of misusers of hard drugs', *Fourth Report from the Social Services Committee*.

Joe, G. W., Lehman, W. and Simpson, D. D., (1982), 'Addict death rates during a four-year post-treatment follow-up', *American Journal of Public Health*, **72**, 703.

Kaplan, J., (1983), *The Hardest Drug: heroin and public policy*, (Chicago and London, University of Chicago Press).

Lazzarin, A., Galli, M., Geroldi, D., Zanetti, A., Croochiolo, P., Aiuti, F. and Moroni, M., (1985), 'Epidemic of LAV/HTLV III infection in drug addicts in Milan: sociological survey and clinical follow-up', *Infection*, **13**, 216.

Robertson, J. R., Bucknall, A. B. V., Welsby, P. D., Roberts, J. J. K., Inglis, J. M., Peutherer, J. F. and Brettle, R. P., (1986), 'Epidemic of AIDS related virus (HTLV/LAV) infection among intravenous drug users', *British Medical Journal*, **292**, 527.

Robertson, J. R. and Bucknall, A. B. V., (1986), 'Heroin users in a Scottish city', *Report of the Edinburgh Drug Addiction Study to the Scottish Home and Health Department, Edinburgh*.

Robertson, J. R., (1987), in *Heroin, AIDS and Society*, (London, Hodder and Stoughton).

Robins, L. V., Heker, J. E. and Denis, D. H., (1976), 'Narcotic use in SE Asia and afterwards: an interview study of 898 Vietnam returnees', *Archives of General Psychiatry*, **32**, 455.

Servant, J. B., (1984), 'Candidal Endophthalmitis in Glaswegian Heroin Addicts: Report of an Epidemic', *Transactions of the Ophthalmological Societies of the United Kingdom*, **104**, 297.

Stimson, G. V. and Oppenheimer, E., (1982), *Heroin Addiction: Treatment and Control in Britain*, (London, Tavistock).

Thorley, A., (1981), 'Longitudinal Studies of Drug Dependence', in *Drug Problems in Britain*, Edwards, G., Busch, C. (eds), (London, Academic Press, p. 117).

Vaillant, G. E., (1973), 'A 20-year follow-up of narcotic addicts', *Archives of General Psychiatry*, **29**, 237.

Waldorf, D., (1972), 'Life without heroin – some social adjustments during long-term periods of voluntary abstention', in *Drug Use and Social Policy*, Susman, J. (ed), (New York, AMS Press).

Winick, C., (1962), 'Maturing out of Narcotic Addiction', *Bulletin of Narcotics*, **14**, 1.

Zinberg, N. E., (1979), 'Non-addictive opiate use', in *Handbook on Drug Abuse*, Dupont, R. L., Goldstein, A., O'Donnell, J. (eds), (Rockville, Md, NIDA, p. 303).

Zinberg, N. E., (1984), *Drug, Set and Setting*, (New Haven, Yale University Press).

Index